When Conventional Health Care Fails You

Simple, Symptom-free Remedies for Chronic Illness and Lyme Disease

Carly Herter

outskirts
press

DISCLAIMER

This Book and the text, information and advice contained herein (the "Content") are for educational and informational purposes, does not take the place of medical advice from your physician, and should not be used to diagnose or treat any condition. Implementation of any suggestions contained in this book is the sole responsibility of the reader. Always consult your own medical doctor or other licensed health care professional prior to making any dietary and/or lifestyle changes and to determine the best course of care.

If you think that you may have a medical emergency, call your doctor or 911 immediately. No action or inaction should be taken based solely on the contents of this information. Nor should you ever delay seeking medical advice or treatment based on the Content of this Book.

Carly Herter is a certified Functional Diagnostic Nutrition Practitioner and a Holistic Health Coach. If you have a medical condition of any kind, you must maintain treatment as prescribed by your physician. The Content is not intended as medical advice, treatments, diagnosis or medical nutrition therapy and the Content should not be so construed or used.

Carly Herter, as a certified Functional Diagnostic Nutrition Practitioner and a Holistic Health Coach has been trained to translate science into practical information, and the opinions shared in this Book are her own. You should always consult with a competent, fully licensed medical professional when making any decisions regarding your health.

This is dedicated to all of my fellow Autoimmune and Lyme disease warriors! You are never alone. We fight together!

To my family, friends, doctors, teachers, guides, mentors and coaches, thank you!

TABLE OF CONTENTS

As I sit here in this dark room all alone, tears dripping down my face, IV's in my arms, fear pulsating through my body, I can't help but wonder, will this be my magic treatment? Will I finally be healed? Why does no one hear me and understand how bad this disease really is?

Did you know that Lyme disease is more of an epidemic than Aids, West Nile, and Avian Flu combined? More than 400,000 people all over the world are diagnosed CDC (Centers for Disease Control) positive every year, but that number is misleading as testing is severely inadequate. What happens to the ones who are misdiagnosed due to poor testing and false negatives? Many have been told it's 'all in their head', get sicker over time, and many are given an alternative false diagnosis such as Lupus, MS, Fibromyalgia, chronic fatigue syndrome just to name a few. One more scary truth, medical care for Lyme is extremely poor, usually insufficient, and in most cases, non-existent in many healthcare systems. Do I have your attention yet?

Hi, my name is Carly, and I'm a Lyme warrior! I don't take that title lightly and I say it with pride! Lyme disease is no joke to have, diagnose, treat nor navigate. I'm a walking, living, thriving testament to that and I'm here to tell you that there is a way *out* of the 'sickness hell' you may be living. We are part of a group alongside over 125 million Americans that are seeking alternative care for chronic health challenges.

My goal in writing this book is to provide you with the information no one gave me. The information I spent years searching and fighting to find. Information that can help you clearly understand what is going on in your body, where your symptoms are coming from, and a clear and easy path out of the symptom-maze that may be overwhelming your life right now. I got to a point where the Lyme was ruling my every existence with pain, fear, and fatigue every single day. But it doesn't have to be that way!

In my opinion, what many doctors or society don't understand is often ignored or judged. That's the times that we are in and that's okay because we can't change that at this very moment. What we *can* change is our circumstances that surround our health, and I'm going to show you how. I hear you! I see you! You are not alone, and my message here is to provide you the hope, tools and experience you may need to permit yourself the most symptom-free, efficient healing journey that you deserve.

My Story

The start of my struggle probably doesn't look much different than yours…

I'm Carly Herter, a Functional Diagnostic Nutritional Practitioner (FDN-P), Certified Health Coach and I now assist people all over the world, helping them find their way out of the depths of chronic illness and Lyme disease… My journey isn't unique. Know others have struggled and have become a success story, and you can too. I'm so happy you are here!

My story is part of the current growing epidemic of chronically sick people, and maybe you can relate. Does this list of symptoms sound familiar? Fatigue, bloating, digestive issues, weight gain, body-wide swelling, joint issues, food sensitivities, brain fog and migraines. The conventional medical community loves to call it "anxiety", but we know it as a black hole of confusion, judgment, fear, sadness, loneliness, and pain.

I was like many of you reading this. My story doesn't start with the initial Lyme diagnosis but I definitely have a series of events leading up to the event! It started at the age of 32 in none other than my dermatologist's office. I had been battling my desires for months on getting Botox injections to remove the first few lines of aging appearing on my forehead. I knew it was a very aggressive drug but also knew many friends using it with relatively no problems...well, at least that they were aware of. They say Botox will help maintain your good skin on top of hiding the lines of course. Insert eye roll here. I ended up going through with it! My doctor relieved my fears by promising that the most common side effects were swelling, bruising and possible eyelid drooping. Please always do your research when it comes to prescription drugs!

Botox has a black box warning that most doctors don't show you when getting the injections. I ended up in the ER a few days after my injections for pretty much all of the neurological adverse symptoms they display on the drug's black box warning disclosure. I've never been more scared for my life. No matter what I did, I couldn't control what was happening to my body. I was having an actual toxic exposure reaction and it was hell for an entire year, at least! And then after about twelve months later, I came out of botulism hell. All was great again, or so I thought until I started to have all these crazy autoimmune issues I'd never experienced prior. Pretty much the aforementioned list of experiences was my new norm, and *still,* my doctors were telling me I was fine. My labs were fine per my doctors. My brain obviously was not. Insert *another* eye roll.

I can't even count how many times a doctor told me it was all in my head and it was just anxiety and depression. I'm sure you're shaking your head with me right now and have experienced the same. Insert smiley face here! YOU'RE not losing your mind, it's not all in your head, and yes, you *may* be experiencing anxiety but it's probably not the root cause! So, I continued with my search. You know, doctor to doctor, nothing really new, just another set of eyes because *one* of them has to know why you're sick, right?! I did try all the remedies though: drugs, treatments, therapy, support groups, traveled far, stopped doing anything…none of it really helped. Some of it actually made things *worse!* But above all, it did help give me answers to proceed on with my journey in healing my body. It wasn't until I completely switched from conventional healthcare to natural that I started to get answers. This was out of my comfort zone though!

I grew up like most, completely having trust and faith in doctors and the healthcare system. I think this can be true in isolated situations but I feel that the conventional healthcare system lacks when it comes to autoimmune, metabolic type issues. If you're wondering why this is, the conventional medical system currently has no resolve for autoimmunity and offers minimal answers for symptom relief and healing. Beyond hormones, steroids and pain management (which can exacerbate many other metabolic issues), they offer little more. More times than not I was made to feel ashamed or foolish for feeling the way that I did based on my lab test results. It truly was one of the darkest-filled, most fearful times of my life. I can say that with a completely straight and genuine face today that **THEY FAILED ME**. They are failing many and I know this because I hear my same story ALL. THE. TIME.

I dug deep into research once I became truly aware that I had to find a better resolution. The drugs they prescribed and their crazy diagnoses just made me sicker, and no answers came out of the madness, just more drugs for the side effects I was getting from the drugs. It was a really, really scary and lonely time for me. I in no way am intending to hurt anyone's feelings. I truly love all forms of healthcare and absolutely honor the role each plays in healing individuals. However, I will be honest in saying, and it might come out loud and clear in my writing, with my disappointment in areas such as Lyme and autoimmune disease care though. This is usually the point that people start calling upon the help of functional and naturopathic providers. Why is that? Well, they most likely have had a boatload of symptoms they've been trying to get diagnosed for years and are only getting sicker because conventional medicine *doesn't* have a drug to fix this problem or the proper tools to uncover what's going on. Or the fact the doctors may be completely missing the root cause/unable to properly diagnose.

There is no drug to reverse autoimmunity to date, and conventional doctors may tell you there's no cure and that you're doomed to a lifetime of disease, steroids, hormones, and pain meds.

This may be true in conventional medicine but in reality, it couldn't be **further from the truth**. I've seen people come into clinics in wheelchairs and leave walking! I've seen the sickest, bed-ridden Lyme patients back to living their lives fully. I've seen people on multiple drugs for anxiety, depression, and digestive aids completely eliminate them and go on to live a happy, balanced life.

My sickness and journey to health have changed my life, my heart and how I view the world. I spent two years, in the beginning, angry and confused, and now I spend my days grateful and in amazement of how even some of the darkest days can produce the brightest, amazing gifts in life!

Once I changed the trajectory of my healing journey, ditched my drugs, (well, most of them) and put my faith and time into naturopathic and functional healthcare, my good health started to return.

My new alternative practitioners did a series of tests and discovered some amazing information that had never been revealed to me. I had Lyme disease, Bartonella, advanced staged Epstein Barr virus, my thyroid function was declining, and I had numerous intestinal infections in addition to body-wide bacterial and viral infections. I had numerous nutrient depletions from years of illness that my conventional doctors didn't notice, and my hormone levels were all over the place. *Of course* I didn't feel good!

I became obsessed with functional healthcare so much that I got certified as a holistic health coach to help assist others out of this nightmare of a maze. I began working with people from all over the world. It's amazing and I never tire of hearing from and helping others with their health journey, and if at the very least, I do what I do in order to spread hope. It's one of the most intimate and amazing journeys I've ever experienced.

I loved my time coaching but felt I wanted to assist my clients on an even more inclusive scale. I'm big on getting proper testing and it was always a downer for me to send my clients to their medical doctors with my list of suggested lab work hoping they would run them, but most of the time they wouldn't! This is why I ended up back in school to get certified as a functional diagnostic nutrition practitioner (FDN-P). I'll explain later in the book what that all entails.

I'm not saying one type of healthcare is better than the next; there's a need and a place for both! Hopefully one day our conventional system will acknowledge the need for complementary medicine.

THE ROOTS OF IT ALL

In my practice, I find that the gastrointestinal system is the most important place to focus on. This is not a new trend as it's been historically substantiated by many doctors throughout history. I also find that hidden GI infections and a toxic lifestyle tend to be the primary root cause of most diseases and chronic health complaints. This book is focused on just that! Whole total body health and wellness.

My typical clients are women between 30-50 years old, and most are challenged with issues similar to what I experienced: fatigue, weight gain, digestive complaints, brain fog, joint pain, bowel issues, anxiety/depression, headaches, and sleep issues. What I'm discovering after running their routine functional lab tests is a common thread: hidden internal infections and an overwhelmed, overburdened detoxification system (liver, lymph, intestines, kidneys, etc.), which are both the gateway to poor health.

My goal in writing this book is to provide a guide on how to re-claim your life, stop living in fear, tools to thrive and education on what is actually happening in your body. Late-stage Lyme and autoimmunity is usually a sign of multiple storms meeting as one creating the "perfect storm". For this reason alone, just killing the Lyme or putting a Band-aid on the autoimmune condition with methods such as steroids, hormones, pain relievers, etc. is rarely ever sufficient enough and can actually be very detrimental. The way most are programmed to fix Lyme disease may actually be doing you more harm than good. The Lyme may not be caus-ing most of your daily symptoms anyway. I stopped focusing on my Lyme and started putting ALL of my energy into everything else. Where are my vitamin levels? How are my immune system markers? What GI infections do I have? How is my digestion functioning? Am I absorbing my nutrients properly? What food am I feeding my body, is it right for me? How is my lifestyle, is it conducive to healing? Am I sleeping efficiently??? **THIS** is my goal in writing this book! There are so many priorities that come before you can successfully work out the Lyme and start healing an autoimmune condition. You cannot continually throw fuel on an already burning fire and hope it goes out. This is the error I continually witness and why it can cause years of unnecessary ad-ditional health struggles and pain.

Our bodies are amazing machines that are very capable of heal-ing if we move out of their way and give it the essential tools to thrive. Sometimes it just takes a new set of eyes and a refreshed mindset to get out of our own way. It's truly amazing what our body is capable of doing if given the proper tools! Healing doesn't have to be so difficult.

There's so much health and wellness information out there, so many gimmicks, so many fads, so many products and programs to buy. I fell into many of them early in my journey! My focus in this book is to strip it all down to the essentials and to help expose the roots to most health challenges that you can feel empowered to address.

I've spent years researching, working with some of the best doctors, trying out hundreds of products, diets, detoxes, and tests, and I'm here to scream it from the mountains: how *simple* and *inexpensive* it actually can be! You don't need to take a mortgage out or dip into your child's college fund to regain your health from Lyme disease.

As Simple as 1, 2, 3...

My goal is to give you the easy and simple tools I've discovered that help restore your health. Spoiler alert: they're tools you may already have right there at your fingertips!

Healthcare doesn't have to be complicated or expensive or loaded with daily medicines for the rest of your life. I've found there are three simple steps to health, even with Lyme in the mix:

1. Pinpointing the "CAUSING" factors

2. Understanding the "EFFECTS"

3. The "SOLUTION" back to health

That's it! It's that simple in theory. Insert partial eye wink. As a Lymie, we know it's never going to be that simple. With Lyme, we know multiple layers are obstructing our view to recovery. We know our journey to health will not be as linear as most. This is why I'm here to guide and assist you by making this as easy and painless as possible.

I've compiled my best information and tools to share with you to help you live a healthy and disease-free life! Let's get started…

Every section is unique and loaded with information I've compiled through my personal and professional journey. **Do not skip sections!** Everything in here is placed for a purpose. Very much how our bodies are whole and should be cared and looked for as a whole, you should treat this tool that I'm providing much the same. We need to know the "why" in order to understand the "how". I find that the more knowledge and understanding I have the more compliant I am to my program and lifestyle conducive to healing and leading a healthy life. Knowledge truly is power!

This is Day One of the rest of your life. Don't let your illness rule you one more day! You can take your life back and feel good and trust your body again. If I and loads of others can do it, so can you. Read on to learn the tools it took me years to uncover and get back to life!

Section 1

The Cause

Numerous things can contribute to disease. Studies show diet, exercise, thoughts, pathogens, feelings, and environmental toxins all influence the progression of disease. Any Lyme-literate doctor, Endocrinologist, Rheumatologist and Oncologist will validate this. If a depleted diet loaded with sugar, lack or abundance of exercise, chronic stress, pollutants, and toxins can cause disease then maybe, just maybe, a nutrient-dense, plant-based diet, daily activity, changing stress patterns, and proper detoxification may help minimize and alter disease progression or even halt it in its place!

I love talking and learning about the body as a whole and how every single cell is united with others in perfect unity. There's so much going on during health AND disease and it's very important to have a general knowledge of the unique balance going on between what you're putting in your mouth to how you're digesting your food, hormone production, and detoxifying the body. It

ALL matters and contributes toward the art of healing!

I think the best way to go about pinpointing the "causes" is to get the assistance of a functional practitioner! You can do it on your own with the help of this guide, a hefty dose of self-discipline, motivation, determination and honesty. BUT you ultimately will save yourself time, money and escalating sickness with a reputable guide and coach. Pinpointing the causes can be something as easy as a detailed phone consultation or as comprehensive as utilizing many functional lab tests to find your nutritional deficiencies, allergies/sensitivities, infections, and imbalances. As we discussed already if every single body system is working together as one unit then there will be no actual one specific problem. We need to identify all offenders and work on the body in a very comprehensive system. As an FDN, I never focus on specific issues. Everything is looked at non-specifically, looking at the body as a whole instead of in sections or parts. How do we do this? By Assessing these core areas of health:

- **Stress:** Precursor to all diseases. This is a priority to get under control.

- **Diet:** Has the ability to make or break any healing journey.

- **Rest:** It doesn't matter how great your supplements or diet is, if you're not allowing your body proper rest, it won't matter.

- **Exercise:** Over-exercising is as dangerous as not exercising at all. You need to find an optimal level for where you are in your healing journey.

- **Supplements:** You need to find the right high-quality supplements for your body. Illness can really deplete the body's nutritive stores, its priority to replete these.

- **Pathogenic Infections:** These usually hidden infections, whether fungal, parasitic, viral or bacterial are huge contributors and often a top priority in any healing protocol.

- **Toxin Exposure:** Hidden mold in your home or office space? Metal in your mouth such as amalgam fillings? These can be THE root of the initial cascade in chronic health.

- **Oral Care:** This is the entry point to the digestive and respiratory tract. Studies do show a strong link to poor oral health and certain diseases.

I'm a big advocate for getting solid answers! I spent years doing trial and error with diets, removing foods or even whole food groups, self-treating, playing Dr. Google, playing with herbs, removing exercise, exercising too much… this can get maddening. Some of it helped, while some of it hurt me over time. For example, leaving out whole food groups can become extremely dangerous to your health. When we eliminate whole food groups without knowing for certain we need to, then we are depriving our body of essential nutrients it needs. I'm a big believer that all vegetables and fruits given to us on our earth are there for a reason. You may not need to cut out all nightshade vegetables; maybe it's just one or two of them. I spent years buying countless amounts of supplements and herbal programs because I knew in my heart that ONE of them was my magic answer. I tried so many cleanses, fasts and detox regimes. Some of it worked, some of it made me worse. None of it fixed the problem though.

Instead of chasing symptoms or guessing what may or may not be the problem why not try adapting this method:

1. Step-by-step assessment procedure that allows you to identify underlying conditions...

2. Correlating test results with your health complaints by the health of a practitioner and validating your recommendations for therapeutic protocols...

3. Potent, proven, professional, drug-free protocols that help improve health instead of just treating symptoms...

> ***"Symptoms are not the problem,***
> ***they are the result of the problem."***
> **Reed Davis, founder of Functional Diagnostic Nutrition**

Our immune systems are amazing machines! This method I use clears most of its healing blocks away, sets an amazing environment, and provides it the tools to fight and heal. Your body can take care of the Lyme on its own. I genuinely believe this to be true.

The lifestyle changes needed are unique to you! This is a challenging area of health that most people struggle with. You may be accustomed to unhealthy lifestyle patterns. Maybe you work too many hours at a high-stress job? Work out too rigorously? Don't get enough sleep or wake up frequently throughout the night? Drink alcohol regularly to offset anxiety or stress? I find an unhealthy relationship with alcohol is one of the biggest contributors to disease that I see in my practice. Do you smoke? Do you avoid or procrastinate physical exercise? Do you eat a poor diet?

Partake in unhealthy relationships?

These can all be major stressors on the body if they continue long term. Chronic untreated stress can be just as detrimental to the body as drinking poison. Stress is now being considered one of the biggest components of disease, and I genuinely and professionally believe this to be true. Let's break down each of these categories and start unraveling where your healing opportunities and potential blocks are...

Stress

> *"Your inner peace is the greatest and most valuable treasure that you can discover."*
> **Akin Olokun**

We now live in a world that romanticizes competition in all areas of our lives. So now, we work longer hours, buy the most fashionable clothes, work out feverishly to have the fittest physique, stay up too late to get caught up on all the housework, volunteer for all the positions because it's too hard to say 'no', shop, shop, shop, go to all the social events to keep up with the Jones', you get the picture. We are all victims of some or all of these occurrences at some point. I know I am! It's part of our American culture these days.

But not all of these are bad, and what's too much for one person may not be for another. Creating the right level of busyness is so personal for everyone. I won't lie, I love filling up my calendar, and I don't do well being static. But when our lifestyle starts to become a burden on our health, it's good to take a step back and reevaluate things.

How do we do this? Well, it's tough to evaluate this on our own. I've worked with several mentors, therapists, and lifestyle coaches throughout the years and they've played a very instrumental role in my personal health. Before I even became sick with Lyme, I was meeting every week with a faith-based mentor. I was feeling overwhelmed in a new town, at a new church, and was a young, stay-at-home mom, and she graciously sat with me at a coffee house for about an hour every week for a year. In our first meeting, she uncovered that I had way too much on my plate. At the time, I was a stay-at-home mom to two little and very busy twin boys, was training for a marathon, had started a network marketing business, was building a women's group, was working with my husband on our family's businesses, and wondered why I was feeling overwhelmed.

She told me that very first meeting to remove everything but my top two priorities. I was like, 'NO WAY!' But I went home and did what she told me: marathon and my boys! I stepped down from everything else. It wasn't easy, but I knew something needed to give to free up some of my life and insert some semblance of peace.

I read a book once that said, 'When we say "yes" to something, we are also saying "no" to something else.' Such a true but simple statement! Unfortunately, that 'something' we often are choosing to say no to is our closest loved ones, our health, and our very own well-being. Take inventory of your life right now. Where are you feeling overwhelmed and stressed? Do you have too much on your plate? We aren't called on to do it all. We are called to be happy and healthy though and this starts with self-care and taking an honest inventory of the stress in our lives. Removing what you can to allow peace and happiness is a huge priority to healing and long-term health.

> *"When you are overwhelmed, tired or stressed,*
> *the solution is almost always... less."*
> **Unknown Author**

We do know that long term stress will impact the immune system negatively. The immune system is made up of a collection of billions of cells that travel the bloodstream. These cells defend your body from foreign antigens such as bacteria, viruses, and cancerous cells. So when we are overly stressed for long periods of time, the immune system's ability to fight off antigens is reduced. This makes us more susceptible to infections. Stress not only creates a hospitable environment for pathogens but it also creates the tone for unhealthy coping mechanisms... i.e. smoking, drinking, and a poor diet. This also escalates a chronically ill state of health and poor sleeping patterns. Stress is a huge gateway to poor health over-all. Stress isn't always an external issue though. Stress can be internal in the form of chronic long-standing hidden infections as previously mentioned. Infections, whether they are parasites, yeast overgrowth, bacterial (such as Lyme and its posy), or viral can cause internal stress which will eventually indirectly affect every single body system.

If left unaddressed and chronic, it will affect hormone balance, digestive functions, sleep, metabolic functions, mood, and much more! Check in with yourself routinely; this will be an evolving practice in your life. This is the other aspect of health aside from diet that we have major control over. If you aren't willing to be honest about your self-inventory, then seek out a mentor, coach, or doctor to talk with and help assess your personal situation. You're worth it!

Diet

> **"If you don't make time for your wellness, you
> will be forced to make time for your illness."**

This is probably the most important aspect of any healing protocol because diet alone has the ABILITY to heal the body! It may take some time but food is *that* powerful! This is a very touchy and personal topic to talk about, though. The majority of our health is controlled by what we put in our mouths. I've read scholarly-reviewed articles in the past that indicate it can be up to 80%! Shocking, isn't it?

Diet is an amazing tool for healing and can also be the biggest destroyer of health. As we already discussed in the section before, food can either feed our microbiome or contribute to destroying it. We need to start taking control of our food choices and stop going along with what we're told or sold to eat. Our food industry is tainted with lies, toxins, chemicals, and greed. It's not producing food for health; it's producing food for *profit*.

Many of my clients have very strong opinions and judgments as to what's healthy or the right or wrong way to be feeding their bodies, so making the right diet changes can be a challenge.

I run many food sensitivity blood panels, and I have yet to come across a client that doesn't have issues with certain foods or entire food groups. Most people have NO idea the symptoms they're experiencing may in fact be a food-related sensitivity or allergy that is coming out in the form of a skin issue, heightened seasonal allergies, migraines, acid reflux, constipation, asthma, fatigue, or insomnia. Symptoms can be very far removed but these are all very typical symptoms of food sensitivities.

These symptoms are all part of the joys of having a leaky gut, which happens in the small intestine. Partially broken down food proteins, or peptides, exit through the damaged villi (finger-like projections made up of cells that line the entire length of your small intestine. The villi absorb nutrients from the food you eat and then shuttle the nutrients into the bloodstream), and your body does what it's supposed to do: fight off the invaders. This isn't supposed to ever happen though.

Food particles aren't supposed to be exiting the small intestine between the villi. This creates internal stress on the system, which in turn affects your endocrine system, which then affects your nervous system (this is in a nutshell of what we spoke of in the prior section. *Internal* stress is just as detrimental to your health as *external*.) Then histamines go out of control and things can start progressing downhill ...and fast!

This is actually the root cause of most autoimmune conditions. THAT'S ALL AUTOIMMUNITY IS: an out of control leaky gut! Your body isn't attacking your organs per se as many may think. It was suggested to me to think of it as a case of mistaken identity, where those proteins that have snuck through the intestinal lining are similar to our own tissues, and our immune system becomes trained to attack them.

Back to the main point... though it may seem counterintuitive, **diet** is the most root-cause place to address autoimmunity, or really *any* health concern. Diet is at the top of the list for healing the body. Food can either be part of the problem or part of the solution! With the food you choose, you're either feeding disease or preventing it. So which do you choose?

Rest

> *"Destroy the idea that you have to be constantly working or grinding in order to be successful. Embrace the concept that rest, recovery, and reflection are essential parts of the progress towards a successful and ultimately happy life."*
> **Sarah Coull**

I think we take sleep for granted. It's one of the body's best natural preventative medicines. Adequate amounts of high-quality sleep can promote health in ALL areas of the body! What happens when we deprive our bodies of proper rest and sleep? SO much bad stuff! Lack of sleep and rest will manifest physically over time. Internally our hormones start to change. When we are overworked, cortisol and adrenaline pump through our blood. If left unattended, it can then create adrenal exhaustion which then affects our entire hormone balance to be thrown off. The adrenals are very much connected to our thyroid, liver, and every other hormone in our body. When this happens, it's common to experience symptoms of depression, anxiety, weight gain, estrogen dominance, chronic fatigue, accelerated aging process, and sleep issues, believe it or not. You can take all the health supplements in the world and eat the best diet but if you aren't taking care of yourself emotionally, which proper sleep aids in, none of it will matter. Sleep and rest are *that* important! If you don't know where to start here and feel stuck (as many times challenges in this area are due to external stressors, unhealthy relationships, financial burdens, substance abuse, depression/anxiety, etc.) then seek the health of a therapist, coach, or mentor. Many times mentorships are free of cost!

Exercise

> **"Exercise is a celebration of what your body
> can do. Not for what you ate."**
> **Anonymous**

One thing to remember in this area of health is that we are NOT meant or designed to push our bodies to the limit day after day. If we are dealing with a chronic health condition, beating up our bodies in the gym will only escalate an already chronic condition. The flip side is also true though! *Not* moving your body is just as detrimental as *too much* movement. So how do we find the right balance for our body?

This was always frustrating for me as I LOVE running. Not just running, long-distance endurance running. This is an auto-immuner's nightmare though, and I wasn't aware of the detriment I was causing or how much I was hindering my recovery and healing time. This became really confusing for me when my body became so ill that I stopped working out completely as I thought and felt my body couldn't handle it. This really ties into what we spoke of in the section above. When we keep our body in a stressed-out state, our hormones react. Over working-out (meaning anything really over 20-30 minutes of high-intensity cardio) produces the same hormones as lack of sleep and chronic stress does in a sense. Our body depends on the push of adrenaline and cortisol to get us through the long cardio session. WE need these hormones balanced to heal from chronic illness.

Our hormones are running the show! When they aren't producing what they should or become imbalanced, every single body system is affected. Maybe you've heard the term 'adrenal fatigue'? This is a common term and focuses on many naturopathic and functional practitioners. So what is it? This is a term produced by James Wilson, PhD, a naturopath and expert in alternative medicine. He says, "It's reading for a long extended amount of time and straining our eyes. Or yelling while enjoying a loud concert and is usually associated with intense stress and often follows chronic infections." Wilson also says, "People with it may or may not have any physical signs of illness but still may feel tired, gray, and have fatigue that doesn't get better with sleep."

There's no science to back this up though. The endocrine society, the world's largest organization of endocrinologists (people who research and treat patients with diseases related to glands and hormones) directly state that adrenal fatigue is not a real disease. I will say that I agree it's not a disease at all. If we look at what is biochemically happening then it's nothing different than comparing it to losing fat while working out. Training our voices. Or sliding into home base three days in a row and creating a bruise or burn on our hip. So, no, I also do not agree that adrenal fatigue is a disease but, yes, I definitely believe it exists and is very real; it also very much affects other organs directly which in turn can create disease. The two major organs that are in direct relation with your adrenals are your thyroid and liver. Two huge power players in every single body and metabolic function. I like to look at this relationship as the Bermuda triangle!

I see this with around 90% of my clients. And rightfully so based on our traditional thinking! Workout more, eat less; you will lose weight. The majority of my clients' #1 complaint is weight gain and the inverse, an inability to lose weight. Most of which are severely cutting calories and doing high-intensity daily workouts to control this. This is a symptom of something usually much larger and not about the lack of working out or diet per se. It's usually something in the form of a metabolic/hormonal imbalance, intestinal parasites, over-consumption of routine alcohol intake, chronic stress, poor sleep, and inappropriate diet for your body. So yes, exercise is completely needed and healthy but reversing chronic illness will require a different mentality over it.

This is one area of health we have total control over. I suggest to everyone that I work with to either cut all workouts to no more than 20 minutes of intense cardio or weightlifting and replace it with yoga, walking or Pilates. If an absence of exercise is the problem then incorporating 20 minutes per day of the same. If you are struggling with adding in exercise, start slowly and work your way up. There are phenomenal free apps now to guide and encourage this healthful and life-changing journey.

I understand if you are challenged with extreme fatigue and body-wide pain while dealing with Lyme or other autoimmune issues; this can seem extremely challenging. I was faced with this as well! I was told during a stress test at one point that my body was acting like that of a 70-year-old. I was in so much pain and so much fatigue that the thought of unnecessarily working out when I was utilizing everything I had to care for my children and husband felt impossible. It did take some time to incorporate exercise back into my life during my healing journey but it is possible, and I ended up feeling better in the long run.

Let's take a look at what happens in our body when we exercise from some of the world's top experts, Neuroscientist Judy Cameron, PH.D., Professor of Psychiatry at the University of Pittsburgh School of Medicine, Tommy Boone, Ph.D., a board-certified exercise physiologist, and Edward Laskowski, M.D., co-director of the Mayo Clinic Sports Medicine Center:

- **Muscles**: The body calls on glucose, or sugar, the body has stored away from the foods we eat in the form of glycogen, for the energy required to contract muscles and spur movement.

- **Lungs**: Your body may need up to 15 times more oxygen when you exercise, so you start to breathe faster and heavier. Your breathing rate will increase until the muscles surrounding the lungs can't move any faster. This maximum capacity of oxygen use is called VO max. The higher the VO max, the more fit a person is.

- **Heart**: When you exercise, your heart rate increases to circulate more oxygen (via the blood) at a quicker pace. The more you exercise, the more efficient the heart becomes at this process so you can work out harder and longer. Eventually, this lowers the resting heart rate in fit people. Exercise also stimulates the growth of new blood vessels, causing blood pressure to decrease.

- **Brain**: Increased blood flow also benefits the brain. "Immediately, the brain cells will start functioning at a higher level," says Cameron, "making you feel more alert and awake during exercise and more focused afterward." When you work out regularly, the brain gets used to this frequent surge of blood and adapts by turning certain genes on or off. Many of these changes boost brain cell function and protect from diseases such as Alzheimer's, Parkinson's or even stroke.

- **Pituitary Gland**: This control center in the brain alerts the adrenal glands to pump out the hormones necessary for movement.

- **Adrenal Glands**: A number of the so-called "stress" hormones released here are actually crucial to exercise. Cortisol, for example, helps the body mobilize its energy stores into fuel. Adrenaline helps the heart beat faster so it can more quickly deliver blood around the body.

- **Kidneys**: The rate at which the kidneys filter blood can change depending on your level of exertion.

So, as we can clearly see, exercise is extremely healthy and needed for long-term health and wellness but we can also see that over-doing it with an already weakened or compromised system can wreak havoc. There are many resources available to aid in this part of your health and wellness lifestyle. Tap into them. You're worth it!

Supplementation

> *"Nothing changes if nothing changes."*
> **Courtney Stevens**

This! This section is SO important. I know I keep saying that but we aren't getting what our bodies need in the form of vitamins and minerals anymore, and if you're sick then you *really* aren't receiving or even absorbing what your body requires anymore. Our body needs assistance when it's down, and what's wrong with helping it in a time of need anyway? What's wrong is that there are too many dangerous products available. The FDA also warns against this as they do NOT regulate this industry. You read that right. The U.S. Food and Drug Administration does not have the authority to review dietary supplement products for safety and effectiveness before they are marketed. The FDA does warn of this danger but also states that "Many supplements contain active ingredients that have strong biological effects in the body. This could make them unsafe in some situations and hurt or complicate health."

There are SO many options available with amazing claims and I fell into this trap for many years! So many companies, doctors, and network marketers selling products for profit having no knowledge or care for the full-body design and requirements. Too many products not really containing what the vendor is promising because of over-production, toxic fillers, etc. How could they though? Every single one of us requires different input! You are unique as your supplement program should be.

In my eyes, there are two main categories of supplements:

1. Food grade

2. Synthetic

There are pros and cons to each category. This section will be short and to the point. You and your body deserve the highest quality products specific to your personal body's needs and requirements (there are a core group of universal supplements that I will be adding into the "solution" section). This can take the help of an expert but do understand this: a vitamin, although it may be healthy and high quality, can become toxic to a body that doesn't need it. Too much of even a *good* thing can be detrimental and may eventually lead to internal stress which can lead to inflammation. Choose wisely in this area and seek guidance if possible.

Pathogenic Infections

"But you don't look sick..."

Oh, brother, that's right. It's time to get into the dirty details. What is a pathogen? Very simply put, it's a microorganism that causes disease. Did you know that our bodies are filled with microbes? However, these microbes usually only cause a problem if your immune system is weakened. Um, hello Lymies! We all seem to have multiple infections on top of our multiple infections.

There are four main types of pathogens:

- **Parasites**- The #1 offender! Parasites are organisms that act like tiny animals, living in or on a host and feeding at the expense of YOU (the host). You will never heal your gut or Lyme if you do not eradicate these suckers. These are too often overlooked. Contrary to popular belief, we all have them. Some more than others. Parasites are opportunistic and will multiply when our immune system is preoccupied for an extended period of time. Lifestyle issues, such as overuse of alcohol, smoking, poor diet, chronic stress, and lack of sleep, can also contribute to a hospitable environment for these suckers. These are so important to pinpoint because they will take everything they need and then some from your nutrient supply. These can be spread in several ways including water, food, blood, insect bites (ticks), sexual contact, and sharing a bed to name a few.

- **Bacteria**- Bacteria are tiny, single-celled organisms that are found almost everywhere. Countertops, desks, your skin, inside you. Most are not pathogenic though, which means they don't cause disease. On the occasion that a disease-causing bacteria enters your body, you can be affected by the bacteria or the bacterial toxin. This is an overly broad category with too many to list but do know that intestinal bacterial infections are *extremely* common with Lyme disease. Common ones that I see and had personal experience with are H Pylori, chronic strep and E Coli.

- **Fungi**- Ugh, need I say more? Yeast is a beast! There are millions of different fungal species on Earth. Fungi can be found just about everywhere! Indoors, outdoors and on our skin. They cause an infection when they overgrow. YOU may be familiar with the term Candida overgrowth? A candida infection is very, very, *very* common with Lyme. I tried treating this for close to a year with little success.

- **Viruses**- An infectious agent that replicates only inside the living cells or an organism. These are the smallest of all the pathogens. Oy, this category is no cakewalk. A huge percentage of those walking around with Lyme also are walking around with advanced Epstein Barr virus. This can really complicate things.

These can all present themselves and be contracted multiple ways and can unfortunately go undetected for years! I've read so many books stating that it's these pathogens that are the causing factors to the majority of diseases in the world. In both my professional and personal opinion, I believe that's pretty on point. I definitely think they play a big part in the perfect storm of chronic illness. I've witnessed firsthand the escalation with my health decline and the diagnosis of more and more infections as the years went on. Because of this, exposing what's happening in the intestines is always a priority at the start of any healing journey. I consider these your 'health blocks'! To accomplish this, a very comprehensive stool analysis is a MUST! Details will follow on this topic in Section 3.

Toxins

> *"Everyone is counting calories when they should be counting toxins."*

This is a HUGE topic to cover! This may be one of the BIGGEST health crises facing us today. Hands down our environment and food have never been more toxic. Many scientists are now considering this as a possibility as to why our children are so sick. Did you know historically our children have never been sicker than they are now?

According to Dr. Leo Trasande, "*We are in an epidemic of environmentally mediated disease among American children today. Rates of asthma, childhood cancers, birth defects and developmental disorders have exponentially increased, and it can't be explained by changes in the human genome. So what has changed? All the chemicals we're being exposed to.*"

This truly gives me chills. We must become more educated on this and do the work to remove as much as we can from our homes and environments. Which chemicals should we be most cautious of and what are their sources?

- **Phthalates**- Personal care products, air fresheners and plastic bottles.

- **Benzene**- 50% of the public's exposure to this toxin is from cigarette smoke and automobile exhaust, predominantly from diesel-powered vehicles.

- **Xylene**- Nail polishes, paint thinners, rust preventatives, degreasing cleaners, cigarette smoke and carpet adhesives.

- **Styrene**- Styrofoam.

- **Bisphenol A (BPA)**- Plastic bottles, canned foods and store receipts.

- **Heavy Metals**- This could be an entire book on its own! Lead contamination could be found in paint and gasoline fumes back in the early 1900s. Even though it was banned in 1970, it continues to persist in our environment today. Mercury is the most toxic of all! We will discuss more of our exposure to mercury in the next section.

Alcohol

"Courage is the power to let go of the familiar."
Raymond Lindquist

I hate throwing this section in here! Insert sad face. I do love my wine. But… chronic illness and alcohol just don't mix well. Alcohol technically isn't a toxin on its own; it is toxic for anyone at certain levels though and creates intestinal inflammation which will adversely affect your recovery or can even halt it altogether. This was one part of my healing that no one, NOT ONE person nor doctor talked with me about removing. I don't think it should be assumed that just because you are chronically ill that you aren't drinking alcohol. It's one of the very first topics I cover whenever I take on a new client or a large cleansing group.

Believe it or not, this is the one thing that makes or breaks the majority of my clients' programs. You do not need to be an alcoholic for alcohol to be a problem for you. It's actually pretty common to find alcohol abuse among the chronic illness community. This truly is one of those lifestyle categories that you may need extra support in. Don't knock this idea just yet! I did early on and was very naive about my dependency on alcohol. Do I think I'm an alcoholic? No. But I did create habits with it that I had a difficult time squashing on my own. I don't think anyone would say that I was a problem drinker; I've never blacked out, usually always the first to turn in or go home, and for the most part, never exceeded my limits. BUT I did find myself drinking wine more often than I should have, especially when I became sick and found the numbing effect quite nice.

It can be exceedingly difficult in our country to go against the grain and not socialize with alcohol, especially when it's SO heavily marketed as sexy, fashionable, healthy and acceptable.

Please understand that getting support doesn't need to mean Alcoholics Anonymous. There are so many different types of groups these days for more than just what you perceive to be 'rock bottom alcoholics'. Alcohol really does need to be removed for healing to take place though. Why is it so unhealthy and disease-promoting? Here's a great answer:

"Alcohol travels from the stomach and intestines through the bloodstream, overloading the liver's ability to process alcohol, directly affecting the brain's neurons, potentially converting alcohol into carcinogens, and taking its toll on the heart, pancreas, nervous system, joints and immune system. Heavy alcohol consumption has been linked to more than 60 different diseases."

Alcohol has been deemed a safe drug but, it truly is anything but safe at any level.

According to Professor of Neuropsychopharmacology David Nutt, who also chairs the Independent Scientific Committee on Drugs, states,

"Alcohol is a toxin that kills cells such as microorganisms, which is why we use it to preserve food and sterilise skin, needles, etc. Alcohol kills humans too. A dose only four times as high as the amount that would make blood levels exceed drink-driving limits can kill. The toxicity of alcohol is worsened because in order for it to be cleared from the body it has to be metabolized to acetaldehyde, an even more toxic substance. Any food or drink contaminated with the amount of acetaldehyde that a unit of alcohol produces would be immediately

banned as having an unacceptable health risk."

It is a carcinogen and based on extensive reviews of research studies, there is a strong scientific consensus of alcohol consumption and several types of cancer. The National Toxicology Program of the US Department of Health and Human Services does in fact list alcoholic beverages as a known human carcinogen. Yikes! The research then goes on to state that the more a person drinks on a consistent basis over time, the higher the risk of developing alcohol-related cancer.

This is one piece you may not be challenged with but if you are, then know you're not alone, and taking an honest look at your relationship with alcohol is worth it. Resources for support can be found later in the book.

Oral Health

"Oral health equals overall health"

If anyone told me 6 years ago that the wisdom teeth my dentist kept nagging me to have pulled out for no real reason were going to be the start of 6 years of horrific health issues, I would have laughed in your face. I put 100% trust and faith in my doctors prior to getting sick; *all* of my doctors! So, when my dentist told me it would be an easy extraction in his office with local anesthesia and I didn't have to have oral surgery to do this, I trusted him. It sounded easy enough. And he kind of talked me into the idea that yes, it probably was time to take them out. I was 31 and most of my friends had this done in high school. I was convinced it was time.

He extracted all four of my wisdom teeth in his office the follow-ing week and it was as easy as he promised. But the recovery was brutal. A week of around the clock Tylenol and Motrin and lots of swelling. Life pretty much resumed as normal after that until I got mononucleosis out of the blue a week later. Mono is a viral infection I'm remarkably familiar with as I've had it twice before. This is more rare than common to get more than once, *especially* in your adult years! Fast forward 1 year with getting a minimal dose of Botox injections for cosmetic purposes in my forehead, and a one-year journey of botulism. Fast forward even more and then a Lyme disease diagnosis. In between those two extremely aggressive infections were multiple health struggles…

I don't know if my wisdom teeth extraction is the sole reason for my health decline the past 6 years but looking back on the timeline and digging into years of research and now being an FDN-P, I do know there is a link between oral health and your immune system. Some doctors claim that the mouth is the root of all disease…

Quick Fact: Studies show that women who have gum disease or missing teeth are eleven times more likely to be diagnosed with breast cancer!

Cavitations, root canals, and amalgams, oh my!

The oral connection can be hard to make. I never had any major dental work done and have been blessed with really great teeth! I've had four cavities in my whole life. Three of them had an amal-gam filling. Then 6 years ago I had my wisdom teeth removed in my dentist's office while awake. I never had any direct correlation to tell me my wisdom teeth removal sites were harboring so much infection that it was growing up my jaw bones…no mouth pain, swelling…nothing. What I did have was ongoing sore throats, sinus issues, constant headaches and stomach issues. I do have Lyme disease so these issues could also be related to that infection or the nagging unrelenting allergies that I've developed here in the Midwest. We have no way of really knowing, but, looking at a meridian line of these wisdom teeth sockets and my health complaints, I was willing to give it a shot and look into the oral journey and its connection to disease. I mean, at this point in my health and the tens of thousands I've already shelled out…what's another couple thousand, right?!

What are amalgam fillings and why are they such a health risk?

"Dental amalgam is a dental filling material used to fill cavities caused by tooth decay. It's been used for over 150 years in hundreds of millions of patients all over the world. This filling is a mixture of metals consisting of liquid(elemental) mercury and a powdered alloy composed of silver, tin and copper.

The chemical properties of elemental mercury allow it to react with and bind together the silver/copper/tin alloy particles to form an amalgam."

Over 40% of the population still have amalgam fillings in their mouths. I think it's safe to say that not many dentists use this material to fill cavities anymore but still, some do and should not be used without caution. They are actually banned in other countries.

This is a fairly new discovery for health concerns and something the FDA (Food and Drug Administration) and ADA (American

Dental Association) does not acknowledge but more and more attention is being brought to the topic from doctors and health care agencies and the evidence is quickly being stacked against them. The International Academy of Oral Medicine and Toxicology (IAOMT), along with several other groups recently filed suit against the FDA seeking an order to require a response to all the petitions brought before them in 2009 calling for a formal ban on dental amalgam.

Griffin Cole, DDS, and president of the IAOMT stated,

"We have banned mercury in disinfectants, thermometers, and many other consumer products…There is no magic formula that makes mercury safe when it's put into our mouths. It's inexcusable to use mercury fillings when there are much safer alternatives."

Dr. Hal Huggins, DDS, MS, was one of the world's most controversial dentists because of his stand on trying to convince the dental industry to stop the use of amalgam fillings. He had been in practice since 1962! He received a post-doc masters at the University of Colorado with an emphasis on immunology/ toxicology in 1990. He was a pioneer for treating autoimmune diseases caused by dental toxins and has personally treated over 5,000 toxic patients. His work included years of blood research to correlate the toxicity levels of patients with amalgam fillings and connecting that with certain diseases.

I have read many of his research findings and watched many of his videos. The information and research he's conducted is quite eye-opening and hard to ignore. Many doctors now work under the training and guidance of Dr. Huggins. My biological dental surgeon in particular. (I will be talking about this later on)

Although Dr. Huggins has recently passed, his work is still being executed and built upon.

So why are amalgams so bad for our health?

Mercury is highly toxic! The vapors of mercury in these fillings are easily released each time you eat, drink and brush your teeth. Research shows that mercury vapors readily pass through cell membranes, across your blood-brain barrier, and into your central nervous system where it can cause neurological and immunological problems.

With a cancer rate of 1:2 and autoimmunity conditions through the roof, this is one area we can control and one less contribution to our bodies' toxicity levels if we choose to get them safely removed. Why burden our health with unnecessary toxins if we don't have to?!

What Are Cavitations?

Cavitation is a hole in the bone, often where a permanent tooth has been removed and the bone has not filled in properly. In the last several years, the term cavitation has been used to describe various bone lesions which appear both as empty holes in the jawbones and holes filled with dead bone and bone marrow. Dead, cavitational areas, which produce pain, are now called NICO (Neuralgia inducing Osteonecrosis). Cavitations are often a result of either ischemic osteonecrosis due to poor blood flow in the marrow, or a traumatic bone cyst.

So in other words, a cavity is a hole in the tooth and cavitation is a hole in the bone.

Who is at risk for these? Anyone with permanently extracted teeth or root canals, regardless of chronic illness! Why does this happen? In a nutshell, most dentists do not pull the whole tooth and ligament out, so the body becomes confused. Typically when a tooth is pulled with the ligament, theoretically, the body will fill in space in the bone where the tooth once was. But, when the membrane is left behind, incomplete healing takes place and a hole with a spongy type consistency gets left behind. What's inside these holes is very troubling and problematic for the whole body. Inside these cavitations, bacteria flourish and deviant cells multiply! Research has demonstrated that all root canals result in even more infectious areas and health concerns because of the imperfect seal that allows bacteria to penetrate through.

Cavitations are a less talked about topic in the dental industry but one that is starting to increase! Cavitations can happen in any bone in the body but most commonly in the jaw. This topic of oral health is on the rise because disease and health epidemics are on the rise. Lyme disease is now more common than breast cancer and HIV combined. One in three will have an autoimmune disease. What is a common thread with all of these? Hidden infections, like cavitations! When our systems are overburdened with infection, whether it's bacterial, viral, parasitic, or fungal, and isn't tended to be that way by nature, disease can take hold. This is, of course, only part of the puzzle but CAN be a big part. As a Lyme disease warrior, I'm familiar with all sorts of infections. I've dealt with parasites, yeast overgrowth, chronic viral infections, multiple bacterial infections, and now cavitations of my very own. Oh, joy!

Does the cavitation come first and then illness or does the illness come first and then the body can't heal the bone correctly? There are some differing opinions on this! Studies do show though that there is most definitely a link between major health issues and cavitations.

One study of cavitation evidence involved an analysis of 112 randomly selected dental patients. The patients were tested for cavitations, with patient age ranging from 19-83 years among 40 males and 72 females. The cavitations were tested using exploratory drilling. Cavitations were found in approximately 75% of all wisdom teeth extraction sites. Another study done by Bob Jones, the inventor of the CAVITAT--an ultrasound instrument designed to detect and image cavitations that have been approved by the FDA and undergoing FDA clinical trials, found cavitations of various sizes and severity in approximately 94% of several thousand wisdom teeth sites scanned. Jones also found cavitations under or located near 90% of root-canaled teeth scanned.

Mostly all dentists and doctors utilizing correction of cavitations and root canals claim huge illness reversal and resolution to chronic health complaints. Many researchers today believe that cavitations and periodontal disease are the focus of various infections which may spread throughout the body and have systemic effects. Medical research has discovered that oral bacteria appear to be very influential in causing various heart, liver, kidney, and immune problems. A collaborative study conducted by the North Carolina Institute of Technology, using advanced tests developed by affinity laboratory, demonstrated the mechanism by which cavitations can cause cancer. Modern experiences also support this theory!

The Journey Starts Now!

It's time to take pen to paper and make an honest inventory of each of these categories. We will be making this list today and putting it into a safe place until we get to section three of this book. The goal is to start really noticing how your role in healing is truly multi-faceted and requires intent and action in all areas of your life. No one needs to see this list! This is for your benefit and eyes only.

Stress: What does this look like for you? Be honest! Is your job too demanding of your time and energy currently? Are you in a stressful or toxic relationship and draining your every thought and emotion? Are you simply not making the time every day to decompress or just be you? Make a list of all current stressors in your life.

Diet: This is a requirement to heal! You need proper nutrition for healing. You need to remove as many inflammatory and histaminal foods as possible. It will hurt no one but yourself to not honor your role in this. Write down what you ate the past three days. Every meal!

Rest: Do you feel rested? Are you fatigued all the time? This could simply be just a symptom of your illness but your body is signaling this physical sign for a reason. Are you honoring your body and providing it the rest it needs? Write down how you've provided your body rest this week.

Exercise: Straight forward here. Write down your current exercise routine. Do you fit in physical activity every day? Yoga, biking, walking, running, Pilates, swimming, dancing…It all counts!

How often are you exercising or not? Write this down.

Supplementation: Make a list of everything you take on a daily basis.

Pathogenic infections: This can be hard to know without the help of a practitioner but testing should be made a priority as part of your healing journey. Functional diagnostic practitioners such as I can help here. If you have the knowledge already on your current infections write them down.

Toxins: This can take some time but should not be brushed to the side. Make a list of your toxic exposures now. Here is a list of ways to consider your exposures:

- Makeup

- Cleaning supplies

- Hair products such as dyes, shampoos and sprays

- Nail polish

- Lotions and SPFs

- Candles

- Furniture

- Paint

- EMF

Alcohol: This is where I see and have experienced my own personal inventory dishonesty. It's time to get honest and write down your current relationship with alcohol.

Mold: Do you live in an older home? Do you have a basement that floods regularly? Possible exposure in an office?

Oral Health: Write down how many cavities you've had and how many are filled with amalgam (typically appears as a silver color). How many root canals have you had? Have you had your wisdom or other teeth removed?

This may seem like a lot to take in. I know I felt that way at the beginning of my health journey but the one thing to remember is chronic illness is really nothing more than a lifestyle illness.

It will take time to create new, healthier habits and hard intentional work to eliminate the unhealthy patterns in your life. This isn't the time to walk alone. We aren't called to do this alone! Utilize support groups, get the help of a mentor or coach, or hire on a functional diagnostic health coach like myself. Long term health really relies on a good foundation! There is support out there to help you through this.

Now that we have discovered what the most common causes of disease are with the stress we are exposed to and creating, our rest, or lack thereof, exercise benefits and negatives, the importance of proper supplementation, pathogens, toxins and diet, let's NOW discuss the effects of them and certain body systems.

Section 2

THE EFFECT

REMEMBER THAT THE goal in healing is eliminating as much stress, inflammation and pathogenic overload from the body as possible. As we discussed in section one, stress, diet, rest, exercise, supplements, and pathogens can all be contributors to inflammation and stress in the body. This is really a simple cause and effect relationship. The goal now is getting into the details of removing the causes safely and providing the body with the strongest foundation to fight and recover. Imagine what your body is capable of if given the opportunity!

The main focus in executing this should always be in the gut. The gut filters and is affected by everything we put into the body in the form of stress, food, toxins and chemicals. This means that if you are constantly polluting it, the gut lining will break down. Very much like a scratch on your arm. What happens if you keep injuring that same scratch? Not much good, I can tell you! Eventually, the injury will start to affect other areas of the body as our body compensates for chronic pain and areas of infection. We don't focus too much on organs that we don't have direct eye contact with every day though so it can be challenging to correlate a symptom with a permeable or leaky gut. It all starts and ends in the gut though and why we are focusing on that area first. You will not heal your chronic illness or Lyme if you don't make this a priority during your healing journey.

What is leaky gut exactly? Basically, it's a breakdown in the wall of the small intestine. This is otherwise known as 'gut permeability', and that term couldn't speak for itself any more clearly.

The functions of the small intestine are as follows:

- Metabolizing or breaking down macronutrients such as fat, protein, and carbohydrates

- Maintaining a healthy gut flora for good digestion

- Absorb nutrients from food

- Help distribute these nutrients to the cells in the body

- The health of your small intestine is a huge priority in your whole health! Your small intestine performs many functions

As you can see, the health of the small intestine is so important! What are the warning signs that something is off here? This!

- Bloating

- Constipation/diarrhea

- GERD

- Gallbladder issues

- Abdominal pains/cramps

- Weight issues

- Gas

- Fatigue

- Skin problems such as eczema, acne and rosacea

- Joint pain

- Difficulty concentrating

- Nutritional deficiencies

- Food sensitivities

Listen up! This is how your body is talking to you. Yes, these are *very* common but they aren't normal, and you don't need to settle for these consistent annoying symptoms any longer. That's your body waving big red flags for you to take notice, and this shouldn't be taken lightly! I could think of no better place to start than here. Well, that and it's my favorite, mostly because these were my priority healing goals when *I* was sick. Folks, there is ALWAYS a reason for symptoms. ALWAYS! In my experience, most conventional doctors are trained to treat the symptom and not investigate WHY the symptoms are happening. When we just treat symptoms, the causes remain and issues can cascade into even bigger health challenges. I see this every day, and I experienced it first-hand with my personal health journey. It's not a fun place to be.

Regaining health is simple in theory: remove the obstacles to health, which are usually in the form of pathogenic infections, minimize stress, customize diet, supplement nutrient depletions and coach up the body's vital reserves. In my experience, most chronic illness cases are lifestyle issues. However, these aren't easy to overcome, which can make the reality of regaining health quite challenging, whether it be a diet that's making you sick, addiction or overuse of alcohol, cigarettes, or recreational drugs, external long-standing stressors such as children, your job, or marriage, excessive working out, lack of sleep and rest, or mold in the home or workplace. These are the most common causes I see in my practice.

These lifestyle issues also tend to create a very convenient internal environment for pathogens to flourish in and for your health to slowly decline. But one thing is for certain, these comfortable lifestyle habits are not easy to overcome and then become the number one reason people don't heal or recover their health. I can tell you this is the biggest reason I stayed sick so long! I had a poor diet (even though I was eating healthy per our American standards), frequently drank alcohol, was stressed out and in a toxic relationship, did excessive workouts, and didn't get adequate sleep. It all adds up over time and creates a poor environment for health.

This book is all about digging into the bigger picture. There's so much to share with you on how to regain your health, reverse your GI issues, maximize your supplement intake, heal your gut lining, and live a healthy lifestyle for vitality.

Whole-body functional healthcare was the backbone of all of this for me, and I'm going to share what took me years of personal trial and error, schooling, and private practice for me to learn.

There's no better place to start than the epicenter of our health and immune system, the digestive (or GI) tract. This is where our food is broken down, nutrients are handed out to various cells for survival, and toxins get excreted. The GI system is doing the most important job of all the organs. We need food and nutrients for survival. If it's not working optimally, then you're not healthy!

The GI tract is essentially a hollow tube that begins in your mouth and ends at your anus. This tube includes your esophagus, stomach, small intestine, large intestine, colon, and anus. The other organs that have real estate in this section of the body are your liver, gallbladder, appendix, and pancreas. The whole purpose of your GI tract is to break down incoming food and absorb nutrients for use by all the cells of your body.

So how exactly does this work?

I'm not a fan of wordy, scientific books but I do feel it's important to understand how our digestion works so that you can understand why it's so important to support. So, I'll make this as simple and straightforward as I can.

The process of digestion starts in your mouth. When you chew your food, this signals your body to release saliva, which helps coat the food for the journey down the esophagus. Saliva also contains chemicals called enzymes. Your teeth physically break down the food, while the enzymes start chemically breaking it down.

Quick Fact: the sight and smell of your food helps aid this process and will actually start signaling your salivary glands to produce saliva.

Your tongue then pushes the food into your esophagus. The esophagus will also then release mucus to lubricate the food's passage through, while muscles then push your food downwards towards your stomach.

Your stomach is found between your esophagus and the first part of your small intestine. When empty, it's the size of a large sausage. Its main function is to hold your food until the gastrointestinal tract is ready to receive it and where the big stuff will start to happen. This is where it starts churning the food and mixing it up with acids known as HCL, or Hydrochloric Acid.

There are many different layers of the stomach and they all have very specific and important roles in the process of digestion. Two key functions of your stomach include the production of hydrochloric acid and more digestive enzymes to help break down your food, and the production of mucus to protect the stomach lining from all the acid.

One special job of the lining is to produce a hormone called gastrin into the blood. Gastrin helps to stimulate even more enzyme and acid production, and also helps to start the stomach muscles contracting. Your food is chemically and mechanically broken down in the stomach during this process into something called chyme. It's a thick, acidic, soupy mixture that is then sent into the small intestine. The small intestine is extremely important!

The small intestine plays a big role in absorbing the food we eat. The stomach actually doesn't absorb anything but water, alcohol, and certain drugs, which is why alcohol and drugs can be so detrimental to digestion and GI health in total.

The small intestine is composed of the duodenum, jejunum, and the ileum, and measures about 6 to 7 meters or 19 to 23 feet long! It's not ridiculously small if you ask me!

I'm sure you've heard of the term "leaky gut"? The small intestine is part of the GI tract that leaky gut is referring to. The small intestine has special structures, called villi, that aid in nutrient absorption. The villi are small, finger-like structures that line the inside of the small intestine. There are millions of them. This is where the magic happens!

They are made of a very thin layer of cells, and these cells allow nutrients to be absorbed into the bloodstream easily. Leaky gut happens when the villi get damaged by too many of the wrong foods, toxins, stress, alcohol, or infections, and incompletely broken-down food particles start to enter the bloodstream.

Once the nutrients are absorbed, the chyme then moves down into the large intestine. The large intestine does not contain villi and mainly absorbs water and minerals. This is where most of the bacteria are found. This is where they're supposed to be!

Bacteria in the large intestine helps with the final stages of digestion. Once chyme has been in the large intestine for multiple hours it becomes semi-solid as most of the water has been removed. This is what we all know as stool, poop, feces, South Park's "Mr. Hanky"...

Phew, I hope that was enough information for ya!

What Happens When Your Digestion is Compromised

Without a healthy diet and lifestyle, your GI system can become imbalanced, and because it's so central to your health, so does your whole-body flow. Hormones, heart function, cell regeneration and growth, brain health, skin and lymphatic system, emotions...everything will be imbalanced if your GI system isn't functioning properly. What drives this? The Microbiome! You're probably thinking, 'Oh my gosh, *another* term. What is that?' Or maybe you are familiar with it.

The gut microbiome is in reference to all of the microbes in your intestines, which technically act as another organ system. This organ system begins to affect our bodies the moment we are born. We are exposed to microbes the moment we pass through the birth canal. Some may speculate we are exposed to them even while in the womb. The Microbiome consists of trillions of bacteria, viruses, fungi and other microscopic living things mostly thriving and existing in the intestines and on your skin. Did you know there are more bacterial cells in your body than human? The most amazing aspect of this system is that it's ever-evolving and diversifying as we age. The stronger the diversity of this system, the stronger the immune system.

So much of what we do and eat can negatively and or positively affect this delicate system. So how do we nurture this system? Well, I will say that diet plays a huge role and aside from that a healthy lifestyle. What can decline the health of this system? Infections, pathogens, sleep, chronic stress, poor diet, abuse of alcohol and drugs and poor sleep habits.

How do you know if your microbiome balances are off? Our body is very smart and it gives us clues! You likely know when something is off. It may be a sign or symptom you wouldn't immediately think is correlated with your microbiome or gut.

It can start small and quiet, with a few heightened allergic reactions, eczema, the occasional headache or migraine, joint pain a few times per month, fatigue, the ever-popular acid reflux showing up more frequently, or your bowels starting to change. These symptoms are all clear signs of an imbalanced system and are often related to changes in your gut health and microbiome.

Though most people don't realize it, constipation is NOT normal, though it has become common these days. This can be a sign of other much larger root problems, like a sluggish thyroid, overwhelmed liver, parasitic infection and or other pathogens, and inappropriate diet for your body type. Or something more acute such as diet, stress, or lack of sleep. Severe and painful gas is also not normal and is a big red flag for intestinal infections and motility issues (movements of the digestive system, and the transit of the contents within it. When nerves or muscles in any portion of the digestive tract do not function with their normal strength and coordination, a person develops symptoms related to motility issues. Quite common with Lyme and Autoimmune diseases). These were all symptoms my conventional doctors brushed off or told me weren't a problem because my lab work was "normal" in their eyes. For others, the opposite can happen; symptoms appear abruptly. This is usually the case in vaccine injury, adverse reaction to medication that your liver can't metabolize, or severe toxic exposure. Mine started aggressively in only one day. I did have a large toxic exposure though. One day I was fine, and the next, I woke up with brain fog, stomach pain, frequent migraines, dizziness so severe I couldn't drive certain days, severe asthmatic breathing, and swallowing issues. It was scary for me!

I had severe acid reflux, so bad that I was having a hard time breathing and swallowing. I was also very reactive to many foods and supplements, although if you ask my allergist, he'll just say it was plain old asthma. He even rolled his eyes when I questioned if food was the cause. Although asthma is very real and needs to be addressed, asthma is typically a reaction to something else.

The Metabolic System

What I didn't know was what role my GI system was playing in this complex scenario of symptoms. As we already spoke of, stress and its triggers of declining health, we should also be focusing on the organ that produces the hormones we produce during times of stress called the adrenal glands. What are the adrenals? These aren't talked about nearly enough in the health industry! They are two glands that sit above your kidneys and have two main parts to them, the cortex and the medulla.

The cortex is the outer part of the gland and it produces the hormone which you're probably familiar with called cortisol and another you may not be as familiar with called aldosterone.

The medulla, meanwhile, is the inner part of the gland and it produces the hormone which again, you are probably familiar with called adrenaline, and another you probably aren't so familiar with called noradrenaline. All four of these hormones are ESSENTIAL to our everyday healthy functioning in the body. They control metabolism, blood sugar, blood pressure, salt/water balance, pregnancy, stress response, your sex hormones (including estrogen and testosterone). It's all about the hormones baby!

These two organs that sit above your kidneys are power players in our rise and decline in health and recovery processes. It's really hard to say what comes first, the adrenal fatigue or the leaky gut, but I will say that you can't have one without the other. Another organ that WILL be affected if your adrenals are stressed out and you have a leaky gut is the thyroid gland. Oy vey! I know, I know. This section feels like it will never end but we have to understand the intricate balance that's taking place between these organs to ultimately do what we need to do and that's to heal!

The thyroid gland has an incredibly unique relationship with the Adrenal glands and has to be supported equally when healing and recovering from any illness. Supporting these glands doesn't always mean supporting them by way of medicines (unless medically appropriate. I have referred clients to medical doctors with certain markers on labs. Sometimes the thyroid does require hormone supplementation.) Although, many times this is not the case. The thyroid usually does very well in response to functional medicine if its sister organs are supported as well and the root cause of distress is removed. What is causing the distress? Testing and an honest health history intake will show. What is this web of sister glands I speak of? Check it out:

- The liver

- The adrenals

- The thyroid

I call this the 'Bermuda Triangle'. Once I really started diving into functional lab testing, I became aware of the decline in my adrenal, thyroid and liver health. I see this to be the case with mostly ALL of my clients with a compromised GI function as well. The thyroid is always the first organ to take a hit in all disease states. I look at this trio like the Bermuda Triangle because they are a trio of mysteries and can become a black hole hard to get out of. IF one of these organs is off, the others are as well. I visited numerous endocrinologists, immunologists, and gastroenterologists. No one acknowledged these organs' intricate relationship and reliance on another. You can take all the thyroid hormones your body requires, but it won't stop the attack on the thyroid gland and the acceleration of the autoimmune condition. It will only supplement the hormones your body isn't producing. You will not heal the thyroid without focusing on the other two and vice versa.

Common Digestive Motility Dysfunctions Associated with Lyme

As we've already stated, leaky gut and intestinal permeability will eventually contribute to systemic inflammation which contributes to the auto-immune fire we so commonly see associated with Lyme disease. Acknowledging where your dysfunctions are in the digestive system is key to moving forward. These motility issues can be attributed to the bulk of your Lyme symptoms. These often go overlooked and will continue to progress your disease if not halted and reversed. The common motility dysfunctions I see and deal with personally are the following:

Small Intestinal Bacterial overgrowth (SIBO)- Which technically isn't an infection, but statistically seen in about 80% of all chronic Lyme cases, and produces over 20 common Lyme symptoms. The small intestine is supposed to be a fairly sterile place. Most bacteria occupy the large intestine, but in the case of poor digestive function, other intestinal infections, and unhealthy lifestyle choices, the bacteria can get trapped in the small intestine, wreaking havoc on your health. The small intestine is the section of the digestive tract where the food intermingles with digestive juices and the nutrients are absorbed into the bloodstream. You do not want a problem here. If SIBO is left untreated then malabsorption of nutrients can quickly become a problem.

Numerous factors contribute to SIBO:

- Dysmotility

- Pancreatitis

- Diabetes

- Diverticulitis

- Structural defects

- Injury

- Celiac disease

- Proton pump inhibitors

- Certain medications

- Immune system disorders

- Thyroid disease

- Pathogenic Infections

What are the symptoms of SIBO:

- Nausea

- Bloating

- Vomiting

- Diarrhea/Constipation

- Malnutrition

- Weight Loss

- Joint Pain

- Fatigue

- Rashes

- Acne

- Eczema

- Asthma

- Depression

- Rosacea

This usually is not tested for unless requested from a specialist experienced with SIBO. Some gastroenterologists are now adding this in but most of the doctors I spoke with during my healing journey told me they simply weren't familiar with it. This unfortunately has been my arch-nemesis! SIBO can get tricky to treat and can take a long time to heal and recover from.

Gastroparesis- Otherwise known as 'Bell's Palsy' of the gut. Just like facial paralysis that can occur in Lyme disease, the nerves in the intestines can be affected and peristalsis can be shut down. This affects food traveling downwards into the stomach. This is a huge challenge to overcome and also extremely painful! There are a few main contributors that are presumed to contribute to this such as imbalanced blood sugar, pathogenic infections, and other motility issues such as SIBO.

Mast Cell Activation Syndrome (MCAS)- This is one of the worst health challenges that go along with Lyme and chronic illness in MY opinion. This made everything else in life so much more difficult! So common with Lyme disease. Do you seem to be reacting or sensitive to everything under the sun? And, possibly, the sun itself???! MCAS occurs when the mast cells in your body release too much of the substances inside of them at the wrong times. Mast cells are part of the immune system and can be found in the bone marrow and around the blood vessels in your body. When we are exposed to stress or danger, mast cells respond by releasing substances called mediators. Mediators cause inflammation, which helps your body heal from an injury or infection. This same reaction is present during an allergic reaction. With MCAS, your mast cells release mediators too frequently and too often. It's so important to acknowledge this disorder and quiet the body, remove the reactive substances, get adequate sleep and utilize proper detoxification. All body systems need to be working together and in balance to overcome this.

There is hope though! I just threw a lot at you, some you may have already assumed and possibly tested for or read about but know that you can overcome these. They all piggyback each other and will indirectly be acknowledged with the simple factors we spoke about in section one. Once you take on a holistic functional approach to your healing.

Food Sensitivities

"I feel like my body is at war with my food"

You may be feeling this way! I 100% felt like my body was at war with my food for quite some time. At my sickest, I got to the point when only five foods agreed with me. I feared the inevitable accidental exposure of something outside of that box. BUT, once I started utilizing a custom eating plan per my functional lab testing on food, guidance from my practitioner, and proper chemicals and herbs, I stopped having asthma problems, ditched my steroid inhalers, and was feeling almost back to completely normal. But you can't stop there because the real question is, WHY are you all of a sudden producing a crazy amount of food sensitivities? You have to dig and really find out why. This is where functional healthcare really does shine!

Disease is never just about the disease. Let me repeat that so it gets ingrained in your mind. DISEASE IS NEVER JUST ABOUT THE DISEASE! It's quite different from an acute ailment like a broken foot. Disease affects the entire body, and it doesn't happen overnight. Cancer grows for possibly years before typical cancer symptoms start to appear. Auto-immunity can take up to *seven years* for blood testing to prove you have an auto-immune condition. Meaning, your body has been imbalanced for quite some time. We need to be doing a better job at listening to the warning signs our body is signaling to us over and over again. Healing needs to be an integrated comprehensive plan. All body systems need to be restored.

The gut is where our body's fuel is supplied and filtered. It's where our hormones are metabolized and produced. It's where our body defends us from infectious invaders we are exposed to every day. It's where our body produces and releases vital energy needed for our day. It needs to be healthy or each body system will be affected in some way.

Investigation of what's happening deep in your gut is crucial for eliminating systems and regaining proper total body health. If you have a parasitic infection, broken down intestinal mucosal barrier, poor diet for your body, misplaced bacteria in the small intestine, poor digestive function, yeast overgrowth, bacterial infections in the intestines you will never truly heal your gut and rebalance your microbiome. This is absolutely a priority in any long term healing plan. Hormones, metabolism, neurologic, digestive all depend on a happy functioning digestive system.

Before long, if not tended to and an increasing amount of unpleasant symptoms can happen:

- Cascading autoimmunity becomes more likely (which is why it's common to see multiple auto-immune conditions).

- Cancer and inflammatory syndromes such as diverticulitis, colitis, arthritis, and dermatitis can develop.

- Toxicity, oxidative stress and mitochondrial dysfunction.

By understanding this vicious cycle we are able to make wiser decisions about how to change our course in wellness and total body health. It all starts and ends in the gut! Let's keep reading to learn the tools to pick up for everything in between though. The next few chapters are focused on the power players in health, our major detoxification organs and systems.

The Liver

"Present actions create future results."

Your liver, the detox powerhouse organ and undoubtedly one of the hardest working organs need to be shouted out here! If your liver is compromised or over-burdened, all other body systems become imbalanced. Both Western and Integrative medicine agree that the more compromised your liver's ability to break down and bind circulating toxins—food metabolites, pathogens, drugs, metals, pesticides, herbicides, petrochemicals, etc.—the more compromised your immune system becomes.

This can be hard to pinpoint and is usually overlooked by

conventional doctors. Not one doctor told me or suggested I should start focusing on my body's detoxification pathways. I struggled through years of treatment, and although some of it helped, I still wasn't living a symptom-free life. I just was stuck at 80% healed and didn't know why. 80% for me meant NOT being bedridden, having decent energy levels, still having food sensitivities, occasional brain fog, occasional anxiety, occasional acid reflux and occasional migraines. This was not a place I wanted to stay. I wanted more for my life! Once I started prioritizing my detoxification pathways, I grew leaps and bounds in my healing recovery.

I always had pretty decent blood labs with normal liver enzyme levels, but the truth is, your liver enzymes do *not* need to be elevated for your liver's role in detoxification to be problematic. liver abnormalities often do not appear in your blood work at the onset of the problems but after *years* of suffering from a sluggish liver. The immune system is the key component here. Without proper detoxification pathways and tools, your body will not heal or sustain proper health. Many people with disease, whether it be autoimmunity or cancer, have backed up or overwhelmed detoxification pathways. The sicker you are, the sicker and more overwhelmed your detoxification pathways are.

This organ has one of the most extensive jobs in the entire body with over 500 essential tasks! The human adult liver weighs about 3.1 pounds and is found in the upper right abdomen, below the diaphragm. It takes up most of the space under the ribs and some space in the left upper abdomen too.

The liver plays a role in ALL metabolic functions in the body.

It is classified as part of the digestive tract, and its roles include detoxification, protein synthesis, and the production of chemicals that assist with digesting our food.

Quick Fact: The liver is also responsible for making cholesterol! While high levels of low-density lipoprotein or (bad cholesterol) are actually bad, cholesterol is also required for building cells as well as hormones. The absence of hormones will lead to abnormal body functioning because they will fail to communicate properly.

The major functions of the liver include:

- Bile Production

- Absorbing and metabolizing bilirubin

- Fat metabolization

- Metabolizing carbohydrates

- Blood filtration

So what can go wrong here?

Many things can go wrong when the liver is backed up while dealing with disease, lingering, ongoing daily external stress, a toxic or poor diet, alcohol (currently the most common liver strain), drugs, sugar, internal stress, long-standing infections: viral, bacterial, fungal, or parasitic, over- or under-exercising, to name a few.

When one or more of these liver burdens are at play, here are some common signs and symptoms of liver dysfunction:

- Abnormal cholesterol levels

- Gas/bloating

- Constipation

- Fatigue and weakness

- Blood sugar imbalances

- Brain fog

- Depression

- Poor memory

- Food allergies

- Skin rashes

- Hormonal imbalances

- Severe menopause or PMS

I regularly see all of these symptoms in my practice. They are actually quite common in metabolic chaos illnesses.

The most common liver problems are:

- Fatty liver disease

- Cirrhosis

- Hepatitis

- Infections

- Toxins

- Genetic disorders

- Cancer

- Abnormalities of bile flow

Luckily the liver is one of the most forgiving and resilient organs, and if given the proper nutrients, environment and assistance, it can regenerate in the early phases of liver disease. There is no machine to do the job of the liver so once this organ is at a certain stage of disease it may not have the ability to regenerate and a transplant is needed. This organ deserves routine spot checks and lots of love. More to come on how to accomplish this later in the book!

Lymphatic System

> *"If you want to go fast, go alone. If you want to go far, go together."*
> **African Proverb**

Yes, this is totally used as a network marketing motivational quote! But that's what I think of when I think of the lymphatic system. It requires a healthy network to properly and optimally do ITS job correctly. Now let's look at the lymphatic system, which isn't talked about much. The lymphatic system is part of the immune system. It's a network of tissues and organs that help fight off infections and pathogens, remove toxins, and remove waste.

Its primary role is to move or drain lymph fluid—which contains especially important infection-fighting white blood cells—throughout the whole body.

Lymph circulates through the body similar to blood, but doesn't have its own pump, and must be moved by physical activity or passively through massage and stretching. We have about 600 lymph nodes in our bodies! This system is made up of lymph capillaries, vessels, nodes, the spleen, thymus gland, Peyer's patches, lymphocytes (white blood cells), and the tonsils. This system is very closely tied to the health of the digestive system, and to be even more specific the villae of the small intestine. The "lacteals" in the villae are a part of the lymphatic system and they pull nutrients and fat-soluble toxins off the intestinal wall. If the gut is compromised the lymph and its white blood cells may not provide immunity or detoxification as needed. So you see how it's never just about *one* body system!

Quick Fact: Your brain is connected to your lymphatic system through your sinuses!

The lymph system is very much connected to the health of our gut and overall health. If our gut is unhealthy or we are unhealthy, so is our lymphatic system.

Signs our bodies lymphatic system is overwhelmed:

- Swollen fingers

- Sore or stiff in the morning

- Feeling tired

- Water retention

- Itchy skin

- Low immunity

- Brain fog

- Breast swelling or soreness

- Dry skin

- Rash

- Headaches

- Elevated histamines

- Occasional constipation, diarrhea, and or mucus in stool

There are many ways to assist the lymphatic system every day! This is so important during any healing journey. A sick body needs help and some simple ways to accomplish this are as follows:

- Drink plenty of clean hydrating fluids

- Exercise

- Dry skin brushing

- Massage

- Herbs

- Near-infrared sauna

- Hydrotherapy

- Deep breathing

- Meditation

- Nutrition

- Gut Health

- Vitamins/Minerals

- Sleep

More to come on how to keep things flowing freely later on in the book.

Kidneys

"A good system shortens the road to the goal."

The kidneys are silent. I don't know about you but I don't really give them much direct thought. One thing is true though, they deserve attention! They do a tremendous job for us every second of every day and without them working optimally we are sick and will feel it in every aspect. The kidneys are two bean-shaped organs that sit below the rib cage, one on either side of the spine. These super-detox centers remove waste and extra fluid from your body and maintain a healthy balance of water, salts, and minerals such as sodium, calcium, phosphorus, and potassium in your blood. You may not be aware that your kidneys also make hormones that help control blood pressure, make red blood cells, and hormones to keep your bones strong and healthy.

Keeping these organs functioning well is key to recovering or keeping the balance of your overall body and health. Healthy kidneys filter about a half cup of blood every minute, removing wastes and extra water to make urine. Pretty cool!

Quick fact: Kidney disease kills over 90,000 Americans every year.

So, what can go wrong here? Plenty! It can be hard to pinpoint the onset of a problem here though as it can start off pretty silent and usually escalates slowly to becoming a full-blown kidney problem over time. Some diseases or other body system struggles that can impact kidney function include:

- Type 1 or 2 diabetes

- High blood pressure

- Polycystic kidney disease

- Prolonged obstruction of the urinary tract

- Recurrent kidney infection

- Heart disease

- Obesity

Kidney disease can affect almost every part of your body. If your body isn't filtering waste out properly then every physiological function is then affected by default. Potential red flags could be fluid retention, a rise in potassium levels, heart and blood vessel disease, weak bones, anemia, decreased libido, damage to the central nervous system, and much more. Let's start paying more attention to these powerhouse detoxifiers, filters, and hormone producers. The road to recovery depends on them!

Colon

It's all about the poop baby!

Lastly, let's talk about the colon, otherwise known as the large intestine! We start the digestive process as soon as the food enters our mouths and it ends in the large intestine, otherwise known as the colon. Technically there are six parts to the large intestine but we are just going to focus on the colon. The colon's job is so much more than just escorting waste out of our bodies. Hopefully, by the time food reaches the colon from the small intestine, it has been completely digested. All of the nutrients that will be absorbed from it have already been absorbed by the body. The colon's main job is to absorb almost all the remaining water and to store the leftover contents until the time of defecation. The colon is a super huge priority of mine! Your bowels are basically a way your body is talking to you. Listen up and pay attention. What to consider while investigating or analyzing your poop....

- Are you having a daily bowel movement?

- Do you have consistent diarrhea?

- Do you have painful daily gas after eating?

- Do you have mucus in your stool?

- What color is your stool?

- Do you have undigested food particles?

- Does it float?

- Do you leave skid marks in the toilet?

These are all red flags! Did you know a possible sign of low bile and specific enzymes to break down your food properly may be indicated in the skid marks at the bottom of the toilet? Mucus in the stool can be caused from numerous reasons…intestinal infections, liver issues, etc. Black stool is a sign of possible bleeding. Consistent diarrhea can be from numerous issues as well, food sensitivities, liver issues, internal infections. I always ask about stool in my initial consultation meetings. Stool gives so many amazing clues! Don't ignore them.

Quick Fact: It can take anywhere from 12-48 hours for the food that you have eaten to make its way through your colon.

The colon gets plenty of attention when I work 1:1 with my clients. I think this portion of healing alone can make or break a healing journey, especially with Lyme, and I'll explain why. When we are sick with chronic illness, our body tends to store things like mold, heavy metals, and hormones and this will contribute to adverse symptoms. The waste that sits in the colon can be there for quite some time and It's my understanding that at any given point we can be carrying around anywhere from 5-20 pounds of poop! Yikes. Now imagine what's sitting there with the poop getting re-absorbed into the body or left there for pathogens to feed on? That's right, your poop can continue to make you sicker! It wasn't until I really started paying this organ attention that I actually started to feel better. It took some time, hard work and patience but it definitely will pay off in symptom relief and healing the body as a whole. Colon cleansing is an amazing tool for supporting the body back to health. Consistency is key here though. Details in the next section on how to accomplish this!

Taking a deep look into the causing factors to health breakdown in section one and now having a peek into the effects truly does put things into perspective. So so so much can happen when we allow continual exposure of causal factors. Of course, this section is limited, the sky's the limit with what truly can take effect when the body is sick! These are the most common I see in my practice and the Lyme community. Identification truly is key here. Not one person dealing with Lyme disease or other autoimmune conditions will have the same cause and effect relationship going on. Every single person faced with a chronic illness has a unique bubble of illness and will require a unique plan out. For this reason alone I think it's imperative to not walk this journey alone and to seek appropriate guidance out. This is where I see many get stuck in the trial and error phases. Don't let this happen to you. We've covered SO much so far! Although I do highly suggest you work with a trained professional, I'm very aware of the high costs associated with Lyme. Insert eye roll. I paid out of pocket over $80,000 towards my medical bills during my sickness. I had perfectly good health insurance. Insert another eye roll. Fortunately, we had the ability to pay these crazy out-of-pocket prices at the time but, not everyone does. I will say though, I still was not recovered after shelling out $80,000!

I see too few practitioners focusing on a full-body approach to Lyme and chronic illnesses. I don't see how it can be accomplished in any other way. Things will still keep popping up and you know what, life is too short to be branded to your Lyme or illness.

Section 3

_____ ❧ _____

THE HEALING SOLUTION

THIS IS WHERE the fun comes in! If I haven't said it enough, I LOVE WHAT I DO!!! If you're really ready to feel better and do the hard work, and I hope that you are, then let's get down to work. Functional health care is NOT the easy route. It's the road less taken because it requires a huge commitment and lifestyle overhaul from you. This is not a "take a pill" and send-you-on-your-way kind of program as you're probably coming to realize.

Let's get down to work regaining your health and back to your life! Don't spend another day settling for an overwhelming chronic illness diagnosis with a hopeless prognosis. Let's turn this around, starting today! I highly suggest signing up for my very intensive 90-day program but doing it alone will also bring healing and recovery; it just may take a bit longer and not as intensive as utilizing the customization of supplements, herbs and utilization of lab testing which is, in my opinion, a game-changer for healing and recovery.

As a health detective, I find the more answers and information we can gather the stronger and more efficient the healing plan will be. The goal is always to achieve symptom relief the quickest way possible. As I mentioned earlier in the book, I'm a certified Holistic Health Coach, a certified Functional Diagnostic Nutritional Practitioner and now a Board Certified Drugless Practitioner from the AADP (which doesn't mean much in the non-medical world but I do get extra training on the daily on drugless methods). So... what exactly IS a functional diagnostic nutritional practitioner?

Functional Diagnostic Nutrition

In a nutshell, it's the study of how the body is functioning. It's a systems-based approach that focuses on identifying and addressing the root cause of disease. Each symptom or diagnosis may be one of the many contributing to one's individual illness.

"Functional healthcare/medicine is the future of conventional medicine available now. It seeks to identify and address the root causes of disease and views the body as one integrated system, not a collection of independent organs divided up by medical specialties. It treats the whole system, not just the symptoms." Dr. Mark Hyman, MD

Our society is experiencing a huge increase in the number of people who suffer from complex, chronic diseases such as diabetes, heart disease, cancer, mental illness, and auto-immune disorders. These illnesses and many more are beyond what conventional medicine can provide and fix.

From the mouth of Dr. Hyman, *"The system of medicine practiced by most physicians is oriented toward acute care, the diagnosis and treatment of trauma or illness that is of short duration and in need of urgent care, such as appendicitis or a broken leg. Physicians apply specific, prescribed treatments such as drugs or surgery that aim to treat the immediate problem or symptom. Unfortunately, the acute-care approach to medicine lacks the proper methodology and tools for preventing and treating complex, chronic diseases. In most cases, it does not take into account the unique genetic makeup of each individual or factors such as environmental exposures to toxins and the aspects of today's lifestyle that have a direct influence on the rise in chronic disease in modern Western society."*

I have experienced this shortcoming in our conventional medicine approach firsthand and it is *infuriating!* I felt defeated, sicker than ever and more scared than I have ever been in my whole life. When multiple doctors are telling you your labs look fine, that it's all in your head and you should be on anti-anxiety meds, but you know in your heart it's not anxiety or depression and that you are truly feeling these symptoms, it's scary, like *super scary!* I don't know what's scarier though, all of these doctors over-prescribing antidepressant/anxiety pills because they don't know how else to help a patient... or that there are *hundreds of thousands* of sick people walking around feeling the way that I did with perfect health insurance and have no actual healthcare.

We work with conventional medical healthcare in the hopes that we can come together to help patients achieve the health that they deserve. I do have to say that I would be lost without my naturopathic doctor and the surgeon who removed my burst fallopian tube when I had an ectopic pregnancy and the two pediatric orthopedic specialists who fixed one of my son's broken arms and my other son's broken collarbone, and my amazing gynecologist that delivered my identical twins! Conventional doctors provide a huge blessing in our health system but we are now finding we have NEW healthcare needs that conventional medicine isn't fixing. Our world is becoming toxic in more ways than one, and healthcare needs are changing. This is where Functional Practitioners come into the picture. We are highly-trained health detectives. We put the Band-Aids aside and use a functional approach to health using comprehensive diagnostic tools.... lifestyle, diet, your personal genetic makeup and functional lab tests to help discover any blocks you may have. We put together your unique custom protocol of supplements, herbs and a personal metabolic diet to help treat and maintain your health so that you can live your life free of symptoms and dis-ease and live it full of vitality!

I've created this program organically through my personal experiences with healing from my chronic illnesses. A few things I've found to be true... The body becomes very depleted throughout the years leading up to disease. Organs and whole organ systems become affected, our nutritive stores become weak, our immune systems misfire or stop firing altogether, we may pick up unhealthy vices to cope or numb the pain and quality of life and personal wellbeing declines. For this reason alone, you can't just take a few pills and call it a day. That's where many have autoimmunity and metabolic type diseases all wrong. Three things, in a specific order, need to happen for long term recovery to happen.

Three phases:

1. Prepare the body

    a. Functional lab testing

b. Diet

c. Detoxification

d. Removing mold and toxins from your environment

e. Supplementation

f. Clean out oral metals and infections

2. Kill and re-build

a. Natural medicine

b. Detoxification

3. Maintenance and recovery

a. Supplemental and lifestyle plan for long term healing

So let's get started....

PHASE 1

Preparing the Body

Yes, you heard that correctly. We need to be preparing the body! This is an absolute must in recovery from chronic illness. I see this ignored too often. It's so important to have a strong immune system, balanced endocrine system, strong clear liver, free-flowing lymphatic before taking on any major protocol. Ever wonder why your body is SO overly-reactive to everything? Or why your "die-off" symptoms never seem to 'go away'? Your body is overwhelmed and can't handle much more! The goal in phase one is to eliminate inflammation and overactive histamine response, equip the body with tools to heal in the form of proper supplementation, minimize major fatigue and body pain, obtain answers from lab testing and start healing the digestive system. We've clearly laid out the understanding of this in the sections above. The body becomes nutritionally depleted, other organ systems become depleted or overwhelmed, the liver may be overwhelmed dealing with too much, and so on. The goal in phase one is to set the stage for phase two. We need strong armor and nutrient-dense soil. Phase one in prepping the body can take anywhere from two weeks to multiple months depending on your level of illness. I always start this phase with functional lab testing as certain labs can take some time for results. Let's learn a little bit more about a few of my favorites that I suggest every single one of my clients uses.

a.) Functional Lab Testing

"The secret to getting ahead is getting started"

What is functional lab testing and how is it different from standardized testing? I get this question a lot! And that's okay! I questioned it too at first. Functional health care is a fairly newer form of health care but gaining steam fast as the need for it is becoming intense as these immune-type metabolic issues and cancer rates are increasing. It's becoming more and more obvious that our lifestyles, diet and environment are becoming more and more toxic to our health.

So what is functional lab testing? Functional lab tests look for proper function and not just disease. This is a key component of health. Tests and ranges typically done by your conventional doctor are looking for disease, while this IS important, disease does NOT happen overnight. It takes many years of dysfunction before disease and conventional lab ranges to expose disease. Functional lab testing exposes the body's dysfunction that can lead to disease. We then utilize this information as a way to support the areas in need. How awesome is that?!

There are so many different forms of functional lab testing available! How do you know which are most effective and reliable? You get the help of a trained professional that not only has extensive experience with them but is trained to interpret them. This is really where you need the assistance of a functional diagnostic practitioner. I've used an extensive amount of them for training purposes but also in my journey to reverse my health issues. What I've found is that you don't need to use many of them! I see this situation abused or misunderstood by many practitioners. These tests are not always the cheapest and many are unnecessary to regain health. I've found that you can establish a really strong foundation and answers with the assistance of two main functional lab tests. A comprehensive stool analysis exposing intestinal pathogens and digestive function and a blood test to expose your body's food, chemical and herbal sensitivities. These two tests will allow for more than enough information to decrease a huge load of inflammation, feed your body the nutrients it needs and clear out your own body's unique pathogens that are causing your internal stress load. Once these two huge categories are accomplished and all other areas we've touched on such as exercise, rest, supplementation and stress are incorporated most body systems will react very positively and health declines start to reverse. It really can be that simple. EVEN with chronic Lyme disease. **I've found more times than not chronic Lyme is more about these 'other' contributors.** So let's dive into these two functional lab tests in more detail:

The Value of Food Sensitivity Testing

This is one of the FIRST functional lab tests that I suggest once I start working with a new client. The food we put in our mouth is that powerful. The goal in any healing plan is to eliminate as much burden on the body as possible. If the food we put into our mouth is 80% of the solution then, this is where we start. Food intolerances and sensitivities may not create an immediate reaction in the form of symptoms. Reactions can be days away, which makes the causes extremely hard to pinpoint. One thing is for sure—food sensitivities DO contribute to the metabolic chaos that is happening in a chronically ill individual. For this reason alone, I prioritize food sensitivity testing with almost all of my clients. It's my goal to assist my clients with doing as many positive things for their bodies as possible. I also aim at decreasing the negative. I find that once people realize how good they feel by eliminating specific offending foods, that we discover with lab testing, the more aware they become of how other things are affecting them.

Food and chemical sensitivity testing are testing for non-allergic immune or inflammatory responses. Testing usually measures two things: levels of antibodies IgG, IgA or inflammatory response, such as a mediator release. An allergy test your conventional doctor typically runs is called an IgE test. The biggest difference between an allergy test (IgE) and a sensitivity test (IgG, IgA and inflammatory response) is that an allergy reaction is caused by the *immune system,* and a food sensitivity reaction is technically triggered by the *digestive system.*

Once I was trained and started researching all the available tests for food sensitivities, I was able to collect more detailed answers for what my body was negatively reacting to. I was able to stop the trial and error madness that typically happens with chronic illness and the desperation to stop or control symptoms. I'm not a fan of cutting out whole food groups, so testing is absolutely essential. Anyone ever tells you how dangerous nightshades are? These are actually particularly important vegetables that our bodies need! Sure not everyone can tolerate them but most can and may even benefit from only cutting out their specific nightshade vegetables that were exposed on the test. There are so many different kinds of testing available for food, and I'm sure as a consumer, it can be overwhelming! They aren't cheap either. And how do you know which ones are actually reliable? Is food testing even reliable?

The answer is yes! I think the more answers you have, the better! I've tried several different forms of food and chemical sensitivity testing and as well as food allergy testing with my conventional doctor. I rely on food sensitivity testing to help my clients recover because food and chemicals are the *primary* drivers of inflammation. The goal is always to keep their inflammation to a minimum, and testing is an amazing tool for quick answers and instant symptom relief. This is a huge contributor to immune recovery and healing on many levels.

Dr. Mark Hyman, one of the top leading functional medicine pioneers, states, *"What works for one person may not work for another. This is called bio-individuality and this is why I recommend that everyone eventually work with a functionally trained nutritionist to personalize his or her diet even further with the right tests."* I whole-heartedly agree with Dr. Hyman!

Food testing helps increase the efficiency of your healing work during a 90-day cycle. If your process goes beyond 90 days, I usually suggest a food intolerance retest because the body often creates new food sensitivities if a certain level of intestinal healing has not been made. For this reason alone, I always suggest clients rotate their food choices as much as possible.

Comprehensive Stool Analysis

Bacteria, Parasites, and Fungus OH MY!

This is not the most pleasant topic but it is necessary to discuss. We typically have not been educated or shown how to look at the *roots* of disease. Conventional Western medicine looks at the body systems in parts: if you have hormone issues, you see an Endocrinologist; if you have digestive issues, you see the Gastroenterologist; if you have a broken bone, you see an Orthopedic; and if you have a heart issue, you see a Cardiologist.

A common shortcoming I've experienced with conventional MDs is that they use labs with reference ranges that are too broad and insufficient to diagnose the true roots of a person's actual health problem; all the while handing out drugs for symptom relief. Too many hands in the pot without enough integration for the greater good of the patient usually fail the patient over an extended period of time. The actual underlying issue is often never attended to, which when ignored, eventually develops into *actual* disease in the body. This can include cancer. This is PART of the reason why we are now seeing cancer and autoimmunity rates skyrocket!

Our environment and food choices are a huge portion of this puzzle but our healthcare system is just as much to blame as well. While ideally, the healthcare system needs to get on board to solve our world's current health crisis and not be so focused on profit and numbers. This is unfortunately a reality we are all faced with. But fortunately, we have more and more information readily available to us than ever before. Inflammation is responsible for 90% of health conditions! Technically speaking, conventional medicine treats symptoms and does not identify and eliminate the triggers that cause inflammation. Functional practitioners work to identify and expose these underlying causes of inflammation and remove that cause.

Once I started looking at my body as one system composed of multiple parts working together, I started to see and feel how integrated and uniformed it all is. Every single cell in my body is completely entwined in perfect harmony with one another. It is truly miraculous! Now it's true we have multiple different major body systems, all of which play their specific roles in balancing our health and life. But, if even *one* system is thrown off balance, they will *all* eventually fall out of balance in direct response.

What are the common hidden infections I'm speaking of? I guess hidden is the wrong term as they just aren't typically tested for.

The most common infections I see involved in my clients' health issues are parasites; bacterial infections such as *H. pylori and E. coli*, Lyme spirochetes and its co-infections; and systemic yeast/

fungal infections; Viral infections, such as Epstein-Barr, are also a fairly common viral infection I've found, most commonly in women with thyroid issues (which came first, the chicken or the egg?). Why these infections are so bothersome is that they are technically gateway infections that lead to other health issues, such as cancer, autoimmunity and metabolic issues.

The good news is that once these infections are removed, healthier lifestyle modifications have been made and the body is given proper nutrient support, health can and usually does begin to normalize. Autoimmune markers start to decline, inflammation decreases, hormones start to balance and more! It's utterly amazing!!!

The body is constantly striving to achieve homeostasis and balance. Assisting the body to remove underlying infections with natural medicine is just one part of the process. Other related supports include supplementing nutrient depletions, aggressive detoxification to assist the body in removing the infections, and lifestyle adjustments such as improved sleep, proper diet, and removal of environmental household toxins.

Of course, functional lab testing is a big component of getting to the bottom of this. I highly suggest every client utilize stool lab testing, as it exposes so much information and creates a much more efficient healing plan if we know *precisely* what healing blocks we are facing.

Much like diet, if these infections are allowed to sit and fester and not tended to properly, inflammation undoubtedly increases and your body is kept in a stressed-out state. Pathogens are gateway infections to other body-system breakdowns. They are a huge contributor to adrenal dysfunction, maldigestion, malabsorption, toxicity, detoxification issues, elimination, and mucosal barrier problems, such as leaky gut.

Parasites alone (which we likely all have to some degree) can create huge health challenges and symptoms. If left untreated, they can lead to cancer and even death in certain cases! This is profoundly serious. Dictionary definition of a parasite: *"An organism which lives in or on another organism (its host) and benefits by deriving nutrients at the other's expense."* Parasites feed off of everything you put in your body, which leaves the body in a nutrient-depleted state. They slowly multiply over time and can be exceedingly difficult to get rid of. I'm in the boat of individuals that look at Lyme as a parasite. I never truly started to heal until I started focusing on my parasite load and eradicating them. My journey with parasites (quite common with Lyme) took eight months of hard work. I wish I had this information back then as it took me a ridiculous amount of time to get past this infection. How unnecessary was that waiting game!? It wasn't easy or fun but completely necessary to get me to the next point in my recovery journey.

If you don't eliminate the parasites, other infections such as yeast, bacterial, or viral infections first, THEN the Lyme will be challenging to get rid of.

Let's take candida for example. This is a common infection in our country but cannot be easily or reliably tested for. For this reason, most doctors do not test for candida problems but treat an assumed infection based on symptoms. I always assume yeast is there in all chronically ill people, and most certainly all cancer and Lyme individuals. This is one of those infections that just will NOT go away if you don't eliminate other infections first. I see too often people get stuck for months to years trying to treat an infection such as candida and ignore all other body systems. They get stuck in a hamster wheel going nowhere but sicker. This is totally unnecessary and could be eliminated with proper testing and the priority of pathogenic infection eradication. I know this well, as I got stuck in this loop.

Healing from disease and removing these intestinal infections *must* be part of the process and discovering what they are is priority! In my practice, I only use the most innovative stool testing method that examines the *entire* ecosystem system. It exposes pathogens such as bacterial, parasitic, viral, fungal that can lead to disease as well as the normal pathogens that can aid in fighting disease.

An article written by Brian Lawenda, M.D., and integrative oncologist states: "Did you know that certain microorganisms hiding in your gastrointestinal tract can cause smoldering, chronic inflammation in these mucosal tissues without you even noticing any symptoms? If this colonization continues for years, these organisms may cause bowel injury, ulcers, leaky gut, systemic inflammation, impaired immunity and possibly even cancer development."

I did MY first stool analysis prior to my Lyme diagnosis. At the time I was having brain fog, stomach pain, overwhelming gas, asthmatic breathing and some food sensitivities. It was exposed that I had a parasite called Blastocystis Hominis (quite common with hypothyroid and Hashimoto disease, which I was told from a very sought after endocrinologist was not a problem for me.

This is common with conventional lab ranges.), H pylori (which I tested negative for on a biopsy with my gastroenterologist) and an extremely imbalanced ecosystem.

If you feel that something still isn't right after meeting with any medical professional, please don't stop seeking your answers! No two doctors or practitioners practice the same. If you are still experiencing symptoms after being told your labs are normal, listen to your body. Symptoms are a warning sign that something is WRONG.

Mark Hyman, M.D. states: *"Your small intestine is also the home of your gut immune system-which accounts for about 60% of your total immune system. The lining of this sophisticated system is just one cell layer away from a toxic sewer where all of the bacteria and undigested food particles live in your gut. If that lining breaks down-from stress, too many antibiotics or anti-inflammatory drugs like aspirin or ibuprofen; steroids; INTESTINAL INFECTIONS; a low -fiber, high sugar diet; alcohol; and more - your immune system will be exposed to foreign particles from food, bacteria and other microbes. The goal is to not only look for infections but also imbalances."*

This is SO much information, I know. I get it. This is a huge missing piece to many healing puzzles, and many times these "hidden" intestinal infections are the gateway to many other chronic health declines and diseases. Intestinal infections whether they are bacterial, parasitic, fungal, or viral they need to be prioritized and worked out for long-term health.

While we are waiting on our lab results let's get down to work... first things first: Your diet! What we feed our body is a way to feed disease or fight it. Let's get fighting!

b.) Nutrition

**"Yes, unhealthy food is cheaper to buy,
BUT more costly to your health."**

We are fortunate in our country to have many options when it comes to food choices. The struggle is what we've been told or simply *haven't* been told regarding what's truly healthy and what isn't. The goal in healing is to gain as many nutrients as possible whilst keeping the inflammation to an absolute minimum. Our food today is over-processed and loaded with more chemicals and toxins than our bodies can handle. We know now that certain foods cause an inflammatory reaction in the body. Toxins, chemicals and inflammation WILL eventually lead to disease. That is plain 'ol fact. This is probably one of the biggest contributors to the increase of poor health, obesity and illness in our country.

Cancer and autoimmunity are disgustingly too common these days. So how do we navigate this if most of what we are being supplied with is basically killing us? This is where I always have to set the expectation and work on mind-set with clients I work with. You need to get back in your kitchen. You need to read your food labels. You need to educate yourself on where your food is coming from. You need to make this an *absolute priority*. Our country has gotten so used to fast food, fast life, fast *everything* to the point we aren't paying attention to the consequences of these options. You too will eventually experience the negative consequences if you don't become aware of what it is you are feeding your body. What you feed your body, in essence, you become.

Quick Fact: Toxins in our environment and food can disrupt our nutritional balance.

The goal in any health journey is to optimize nutrient intake and to decrease inflammation and histamines. With that said, you then need to make some major eliminations *and fast*. When working with me, it is mandatory to cut out ALL gluten and animal dairy sources during the healing process. Why? They cause inflammation, mucus production and usually some level of a histamine reaction. Remember, the goal to heal is to eliminate those three burdens. This is something we have control over and a way to support the body. It's truly an amazing tool!

Our gluten and animal dairy is not the same as it used to be back in the day, unfortunately. So what makes them different now? They're typically filled with chemicals and over-processed to the point where our bodies respond to them as toxins in our systems. They usually create damage and inflammation in even the healthiest of bodies! These are the two biggest offenders I start eliminating with my clients. Dairy doesn't agree with most people! According to the National Digestive Diseases Information Clearinghouse, some 30 to 50 million Americans are lactose intolerant, including up to 75% of African Americans and American Indians and 90% of Asian Americans. Although, these stats don't seem alarming considering there are 330 million people in America! After looking through months of peer-reviewed scientific studies to back-up everything I'm saying here I couldn't find one peer-reviewed scientific study, NOT ONE to back this up! I was shocked! After years of listening to podcasts, professors, doctors claiming how dangerous it can be, I was floored to find no actual scientific peer-reviewed back-up. I have my suspicions about why, yet nonetheless, there are boatloads of literature, doctors, and schools that will state how toxic, inflammatory and histamine causing our animal dairy CAN be. As well as an ever-evolving American dietary food pyramid. My solution to this is to try this for yourself! My clients are usually amazed at how good they feel after completely eliminating animal dairy. ***That's all the proof you need!***

The FDA also reports these same statistics as stated above and goes on to further explain the difference between a lactose allergy and a lactose sensitivity (which the majority of the population seems to fall under). Amena Warner, the head of clinical services at Allergy UK exclaims, "Intolerances are different from food allergies; they are not caused by the immune system and are not life-threatening." Milk allergy is the second most common food allergy after peanuts! A milk allergy is far more common in young children and infants, while intolerance typically affects adults. Why? Per the FDA, "as people age their bodies produce fewer lactase enzymes" Lactase is the enzyme that breaks down lactose, which is the sugar found in dairy.

Gluten has been clinically proven to cause damage in even non-gluten sensitive people who show no symptoms per Dr. Alessio Fasano of Harvard, the world's top gluten expert. Well, if you're anything like me, I had a hard time digesting this information at first. Gluten products have been around for decades! It's actually a 10,000-year-old food tradition. But, in the last few generations, things have changed. Why all of a sudden is it now bad? I dug deep on this topic to help you understand more scientifically why so many are struggling with our food and in particular our gluten products. Many opinions are being thrown around online about this, but once you go gluten-free and physically feel the difference in your body, you may side more with the stacking evidence on just how bad gluten-containing products are for your long term health. Studies proving this are as follows:

1. PubMed.gov: Nutritional wheat amylase-trypsin inhibitors promote intestinal inflammation via activation of myeloid cells.

2. PubMed.gov: Wheat Amylase trypsin inhibitors drive intestinal inflammation via activation of toll-like receptor 4.

3. PubMed.gov: Wheat amylase trypsin inhibitors as nutritional activators of innate immunity.

4. PubMed.gov: Wheat amylase-trypsin inhibitors exacerbate intestinal and airway allergic immune responses in humanized mice.

5. PubMed.gov: Non-coeliac gluten sensitivity- A new disease with gluten intolerance.

6. PubMed.gov: Gluten Sensitivity.

7. PubMed.gov: High prevalence of celiac disease in patients with lactose intolerance.

8. Ncbi.nlm.nih.gov: Spectrum of gluten-related disorders: Consensus on new nomenclature and classification.

9. Scirp.org: Cross-reaction between gliadin and different food and tissue antigens.

10. PubMed.gov: Non-celiac wheat sensitivity: differential diagnosis, triggers and implications.

I will stop there, but please do investigate these peer-reviewed biomedical literature pieces on how inflammatory causing gluten, wheat and grains are for not just chronically ill individuals but most people. And, if you still seem skeptical, then attempt a gluten-free diet for 30 days and enjoy the many physical benefits! That will be all the proof you need.

Some simple actions you can take to re-empower your relationship with food include:

- Growing a vegetable garden

- Visiting your weekly farmers' market

- Simply ditching all the inside aisles at the grocery store and focusing on produce and organic meat in the outside aisles

- Getting back in the kitchen and starting to make everything from scratch

Statistics currently show that 1 in 2 people will get cancer in their lifetime, 1 in 4 will die from it, and 1 in 3 will get an autoimmune disease. How terrifying. AND *diet* plays a major role in this!

If you think you don't have the time to get back in the kitchen and ditch the processed and fast foods, I invite you to think of how much developing an illness or sickness would take from your life.

Rearranging your diet can take some getting used to but anything can be made a habit, and bad habits, such as eating out 5 nights per week or relying on store-bought, prepared foods, *can* be broken. I was once that girl. I love dining out! It's easy, fun, and social. But the consequences will never be worth it. How would you feel if you learned you contributed to your own illness and potentially your own...*death?*

But once I got sick, I slowly learned how terrible consuming processed foods made me feel and contributed to my symptoms. For example, once I started digging deeper, I slowly started to realize my diagnosed asthma wasn't actually "asthma" at all! What I had was major food sensitivities and allergies that were causing my asthmatic breathing.

Once I kicked the high-histamine and offending foods to the curb, my digestion improved, my breathing normalized, migraines disappeared, sleep improved, brain fog diminished, mood improved, and so much more. It is quite miraculous how a simple food lifestyle change can positively impact your health and quality of life. We are going for vitality and longevity here people!

What I Recommend Eating

I'm not a fan of specific diets. I don't adhere to Paleo, Keto, Whole 30, or 21-day-fix types of eating plans. I've tried them all and then some, and although they're great, they don't work for everyone. No matter who you are, where you come from and what your genetic makeup is, they are simply not sustainable long-term and not effective for everyone. Diets are not a one-size-fits-all, so we should stop approaching them as if they are! We all have too many differences and chemical makeups to have any of these diet trends make sense.

So what exactly DOES work you may be asking? Well, no worries; there is an answer! The goal with your diet is to always eat as many nutrient-dense and appropriate foods as possible to keep healing and recovery at the forefront of your eating priorities.

Here's what I suggest:

- 80% of your plate should be a mixture of organic vegetables

- 10% organic, plant-based starches

- 10% easily digestible animal or seafood proteins

- Fill-ins on every plate: plant-based, unsweetened, organic dairy, and seeds; and high-quality unsaturated fats: coconut oil, olive oil, avocados, olives

You may realize several key factors are missing from this list. They are:

- Animal dairy

- Wheat/gluten products

- Corn

- Soy

- Processed sugar

- Alcohol

Large quantities of sugar, by the way, are present in basically ALL processed foods. Sugar is now being defined as one of the biggest inflammatory-causing food additives of all times and we usually consume *way* too much sugar in our diets. Now let's break down our plate even more and look at one area of our food that contributes to some very harsh symptoms of illness...

Histamine And How It Affects Your Health

What is histamine and why should you focus on this? Histamine is a neurotransmitter and immune modulator which can be involved in the dysregulation of immune, digestive, and central nervous system function. You might not give histamine a second thought. To most people, it's a seasonal allergy issue. But what many don't realize is that high-histamine foods or your personal offending foods and or chemicals may be a huge contributor to your chronic illness and/or symptoms. Thousands of peer-reviewed studies point to this!

This portion alone will often make or break someone's recovery or long-term health success. The histamine-producing products—whether herbs, medications, or foods—need to be removed and or dramatically reduced for inflammation and/or symptoms to resolve.

Histamine isn't a bad thing though. This is one of the many ways our body talks to us to tell us something is wrong. Technically speaking, histamine causes our blood vessels to swell or dilate so that your white blood cells can quickly find and attack the infection or problem. The build-up of histamine is what creates the headache, hives, eczema, fatigue, body pain, itchy eyes, or throat.

If the goal and plan are to heal, then this is a particularly important aspect of eating that needs to be prioritized. While in recovery mode I suggest eliminating top histamine producing foods such as:

- Egg Whites

- Shellfish

- Cured meats

- Canned fish

- Beer and red wine

- Nuts

- Animal dairy

- Gluten

Quick Fact: About 90% of all food allergies are caused by seven foods: dairy, soy, shellfish, wheat, gluten, peanuts, and egg whites.

Creating a highly nutritious, low-histamine diet is one of the biggest gifts you can give to your body while it heals.

Let's break down our plate even more now! We need a good balance of micro and macronutrients to properly feed our cells. Micronutrients are vitamins, minerals, trace elements, phytochemicals, and antioxidants. Macronutrients are the energy-giving, caloric components of our food that most of us are familiar with: carbohydrates, fats, and proteins.

In Western culture, we are used to big, fast meals that may include pizza with lots of cheese, or sitting down to a big, juicy burger and bun loaded with cheese with a side of fries, or a breakfast completely made of sugar in the form of cereal or baked goods like muffins. When we eat just to please our taste buds (because let's be honest, a big juicy burger on a delicious sesame seed bun topped with cheese, bacon and mayo with a side of fries IS absolutely delicious) then we place our health as a second priority. It just isn't the most nutrient-dense meal, and that is what we should be striving for.

Every meal should be an opportunity to feed your body what it needs to run properly and healthfully. Let's examine breakfast for another example. Our typical American standard go-to food is a baked good, cereal, breakfast bar, smoothie loaded with all fruit, or processed yogurt (which is mostly sugar). Are these options we've become accustomed to beginning our day with nutrient-based? When we choose a nutrient *lacking* breakfast to begin our day, we ultimately start our day on a deficit.

We need to be overhauling our food choices. In my opinion, there's no better breakfast option than a freshly made egg yolk scramble with vegetables, raw juice loaded with vegetables, or a cup of vegetable soup! Our body wants us to start our day feeding it the nutrients it needs, and NOT foods composed of mostly sugar and empty calories.

Let me explain even further. Junk foods that are causing inflammatory or histamine reactions in your body create internal stress, which can create the symptoms I've mentioned: bloating, migraines, brain fog, digestive problems, sleeping issues, joint pain, hormone imbalance, and more. These are the typical symptoms many autoimmune, Lyme, and chronic-illness patients complain of. And this can start even at your first meal of the day!

These are typically signs that histamine, hormones, and

inflammation are running rampant in the body. Cutting out the offending foods creates space and energy for your body to do what it needs to do: rebalance, decrease inflammation, and heal.

Food is immensely powerful! This is one piece that we have control over. Food can make an already sick person sicker or help to relieve symptoms. And sometimes to complete remission!

Adopting an anti-inflammatory/histamine diet that is right for you is your biggest homework during treatment and recovery!

c.) Detoxification

> *"While detox diets don't do anything that your body can't naturally do on its own, you can optimize your body's natural detoxification system."*

When we are sick for long periods of time, our detoxification organs such as the lymphatic system and the liver really take a big hit and can become overwhelmed and backed up. This is the part of my health habits and my nutrition practice that I'm most passionate about. This one piece of your health can make or break your recovery!

WHY IT'S SO IMPORTANT TO DETOX *REGULARLY*

The human body is a self-healing, self-renewing, self-cleansing organism. When the right conditions are created, vibrant well-being is its natural state. We have departed from the ways of nature and live under less-than-natural conditions!

Like global warming, the toxicity of our planet is undeniable. The air we breathe, the water we drink and shower with, the foods we eat, the cosmetics we use, and the buildings we live and work in are loaded with toxic chemicals that alone or in combination cause disease, suffering, and even death.

When we remove these obstacles and add what is lacking such as whole natural foods, a lifestyle conducive to healing, high-quality sleep, proper exercise, nutrients, our bodies bounce back into health as if by magic. This is natural, common-sense medicine, enabling the body to heal, regenerate and even heal itself.

We live in an overly chemical world that is loaded with toxins. Our food, water, air, soil, drugs, and fast-paced, money-driven lifestyles all overburden our body systems. Detoxification is how our bodies get all this muck cleaned up. Fortunately, our bodies possess self-regulating healing mechanisms. A healthy body is capable of eliminating toxic substances. The challenge starts happening when the production of toxic metabolites and the ingestion of toxic substances overwhelms the organs of detoxification. This is typical of chronic illnesses! The body stores these substances in the connective tissues which then impedes their important tasks. Support in this area is so important during illness when our whole system becomes overburdened. Toxins leave via your urine, stool, breath, and sweat.

As we discussed above, there are *many* different organs and functions that take place or have a role in detoxifying toxins out of our system, and they are all equally important in this delicate balance to keep us healthy. We will be discussing many ways to detoxify the body. Let's start with the colon...

My favorite ways to accomplish colon detoxification include:

- Herbs

- Professional colonics

- Coffee enemas

- Salt flushing

My personal favorite is the salt flush. This is not as crazy as it sounds and actually appears to be safer than many commercial-grade colon-cleansing drugs, laxatives, teas, or diuretics per Dr. Josh Axe.

> *"The fact is that for many people-especially those eating poor diets-toxins, heavy metals and waste build up in the colon over time due to digestive issues and can contribute to inflammation, low energy and possibly even disease development. A salt water flush is a safe, simple and effective way to clear things out entirely now and then."*
> **Dr. Josh Axe.**

Let's turn this question around. Is it safe to stay sick? No. A very big NO! Sickness, if not dealt with properly, leads to further sickness.

Although this seems out of the box and totally unnecessary, I've found that when challenged with a chronic illness, the body is overburdened with too much. Too much stress, toxins, pathogenic infections, hormonal imbalances and much more per what we've already covered in section 1. The goal is to eliminate the body's burden. This method is just another tool in our toolbox to accomplish this.

When I was at my sickest, I couldn't tolerate even a single vitamin supplement. Every protocol I was taking orally I was reacting with severe reactions like brain fog, breathing difficulty, severe stomach pain, spine pain, dizziness, sleeplessness…you may be experiencing some of the same? Please know that your body is just overburdened and it just needs to be assisted a bit.

This is only one of the many effective ways to support the healing process. Salt flushing serves so many different purposes and costs little to no money at all. The goal with the salt flush is to empty the colon, clear out some pathogens, yeast, and purge out extra mucus, much like sinus irrigation. Not only that but many of us are actually *deficient* in the essential minerals found in sea salt. Sea salt is very different from table salt. DO NOT USE TABLE SALT FOR THIS DETOXIFICATION! Expect to be in the bathroom clearing out your colon for a good hour and be sure to drink lots of water throughout the day. Here is how you do a salt flush detox (also see disclaimer below before trying a new detox):

Salt Flushes are something I do first thing in the morning on an empty stomach. I mix 1 tablespoon of really good, fine-grained mineral sea salt, with two cups of lukewarm water and squeeze in half a lemon. Drink this very fast and quickly follow it up with a few cups of room temperature water. Lay on your left side and massage your belly in a clockwise motion. This will get things moving. I suggest doing this two times per week for four weeks and then decreasing to once per week for the remainder of your healing journey.

Disclaimer: I absolutely LOVE salt flushing but do this detox ONLY if you're adhering to a very plant-based, whole food diet. If you are eating a regular diet of processed high sodium foods, this would not be the time to try this, as well as if you have high blood pressure and are pregnant or going through cancer treatment. And of course, ALWAYS consult with your doctor if you're unsure.

Herbs are another amazing tool to accomplish this. No need to buy expensive herbal programs. Some very unique and time-tested powerhouse herbs are super inexpensive, such as cascara sagrada, senna and flaxseed. If you are finding yourself super reactive to herbal mixtures, then buy yours individually from a reputable vendor. This is what I did for a few months during my sickest times.

Coffee enemas are quite efficient but not everyone can tolerate them. A coffee enema is a really great way to nudge the liver to purge unnecessary toxins, hormones and pathogens. These can also be fairly inexpensive! I usually only suggest these at a certain level of healing such as once your diet is under control and high-quality rest and sleep are happening as well as if your food sensitivity testing doesn't expose coffee as a dietary offender. Many are shocked to find that they are quite reactive to it.

Professional Colonics is not my jam but people do love them! I'm not a fan of sitting in front of someone else cleaning out my rear. Insert emoji scrunchy face. It does get the job done though, and all without having to mess with anything at home yourself... which is also an interesting experience!

Other amazing methods of detoxification which should be incorporated in addition to regularly clearing out the colon include:

- Epsom salt baths

- Dry skin bruising

- Lymphatic massage

- Hot or cold therapy

- Ball bouncing (otherwise known as rebounding)

- Light exercise

THIS SECTION IS SO IMPORTANT! During chronic illness, the body may accumulate toxic waste that needs to be removed from our body. Detoxification should be a full-time job until symptoms resolve. This can take months! I utilized a salt flush daily for almost eight months. I was also incorporating bimonthly lymphatic massages, yoga, Epsom salt baths a few nights per week and dry skin brushing. If you are unfamiliar with dry skin brushing (as I was) It's truly amazing and I highly suggest giving it a try. I like to do this no more than twice per week. Using a natural bristle brush, gently but firmly brush your skin in long strokes toward your heart, going over each area a few times. This is typically done prior to showering and I always follow it up with a really good food-grade massaging oil. Assisting the body in this way will only speed the process of healing. The removal of metabolic waste will assist in alleviating the toxic burden we've taken on during illness. Benefits of doing this include reduced toxic load, better energy, sleep, digestion, mood and overall sense of wellbeing, which all aids in your healing process!

Environmental Detoxification

Yes, you read that right. We need to clean up our homes and what we are putting on our bodies. This is just as important as everything else. DO NOT skip this step or think it's not a problem for you. *Every single* toxin we expose ourselves to is adding to our health decline.

Ways Your Body Is Exposed to Toxins:

- Air and water pollution

- Clothing

- Building materials and furnishings

- Food additives

- Medications

- Radiation

- Cosmetics and toiletries

- Household cleaners

- Alcohol

- Insecticides and pesticides in food

- Chemicals, including aluminum and mercury in vaccines

- Heavy metals in the environment, in foods, and from

occupational exposure

- Stress

- Excess sugar

It's time to take a look at this list and make an honest personal inventory of it all in your own life. It's now time to take out that list we made back in section 1!

This step could easily be overlooked or brushed aside. Please do not do that! Detoxing the air you breathe and expose your skin to on a daily basis is equally as important as everything else we've touched upon here so far. We get used to our products, cleaning, beauty, furniture…etc. We trust the companies selling them to us because they have to follow health standards, right? I've found this to be furthest from the truth!

This is where you need to really become your own advocate. A friend mentioned to me a few years back, after the annoyance of a conversation of chemicals in our processed foods, 'When does it stop?' It can become maddening having to put this amount of work into our health! It's true. WE have to do the work to protect our long-term health. Certain chemicals in cleaning products have been linked to fertility problems, birth defects, increased risks of breast cancer, asthma, hormone disruption, and much more. There is no regulation around this industry requiring companies to list all the ingredients in the products. Which means companies can keep toxic chemicals a secret from you. AHHH! The very bottom line here is that there shouldn't be any toxic ingredients in the products we are using to clean our homes. Come on.

To add insult to injury, I recently read that only 4% of women think they are beautiful. That's so very sad to me, but also, I've noticed many women feel the need to keep buying more and more beauty products. The beauty industry knows this and markets it to our very insecurities. The average woman puts over *500 toxins* on her skin every day, and of that horrific number, *60%* is absorbed into her skin. This only contributes to our toxic burden! Insert sad face.

Luckily the beauty industry is starting to acknowledge how dangerous our products have become and newer, high-quality brands are now popping up! Of course like anything, some of them are also plain bad and poor performing, but lucky for you I've been trying them for years and my favorite high performing lines are as follows:

- Beauty Counter

- Honest Company

- Juice Beauty

- 100% Pure Beauty

- Kjaer Weis

Hair, skin, makeup…and it doesn't stop there.

While on the topic of toxins, let's also talk about alcohol! This is a major toxin that has not only been socially normalized but also branded by the media as healthy. This is anything but that and needs to be eliminated for the healing of disease. As we mentioned earlier, there are no safe amounts and the FDA keeps adjusting safe limits for health because of new research coming forward. The most effective action step here is complete removal until complete healing has taken place. Meaning, no symptoms for 6 months (my personal gage and opinion). If you are struggling with this and not identifying as an alcoholic (many are not, some may be just caught up in a grey area of drinking) then some amazing alternatives are as follows:

- Sobersis: An online women-only Christian-focused group to assist women who are seeking a sober-minded life. A group that focuses on the role of drinking with a holistic approach.

- Ditched the Drink: A wellness coach offering online closed group support.

- Annie Grace: Author of This Naked Mind, and guide of many online support groups for removing alcohol.

- Celebrate Recovery

- Smart Recovery

There are SO many more options such as amazing podcasts, books, influencers, and bloggers. I've utilized all of these options at different times during my healing journey and highly recommend all of them! This is a movement that is quickly picking up steam! So many yummy alcohol-free beverages, mocktails and spirit-free bars are becoming available now.

Our cleaning products are very dangerous! The most toxic room in the house is surprisingly the laundry room. With three small kids, I spend a good chunk of my week in this room folding and washing. An easy swap out here is ensuring you have good ventilation and safer products. Think about how often you clean your countertops in the kitchen, light a candle to fragrance the smell of the room, mop your floor, possibly breathing in mold hiding in the walls? All of this adds up every single day! BUT HAVE NO FEAR! There are so many cleaner brands on the market. Take Vinegar for example. It's always a safe, inexpensive and very effective go-to for cleaning just about anything in the house if you're overwhelmed with options or the cost. My store-bought safer alternatives are as follows:

- Mrs. Meyers

- Seventh Generation

- Honest Brand

- Branch Basics

- Aunt Fannies

- Better Life

- Dr. Bronners

Try to think past the fake fragrant smells you've become used to and put safer products as a priority. Try to get the whole family on board with your home detoxification!

d.) Mold

"All I want is a clear mind and a happy heart."

Mold should also be a top priority in clearing your home and your body! Mold could be THE very culprit to all of your health issues. This sneaky little devil definitely deserves an entire section dedicated to it. Mold is sly and can be found even in the most unexpected of places in the home and office. If you're dealing with Lyme, you are most likely familiar with mold toxicity and its role in your illness. It just seems to go hand-in-hand with Lyme disease.

Dr. Wayne Anderson, ND states, *"The medical community has generally underappreciated its effects upon the brain and immune system. Mold affects the entire body in the same way as bacterial infections. The toxins stick to the surface of the cells and are absorbed into the cells, where they cause inflammation and cellular dysfunction."* He goes on to then say that *"Lyme and mold affect the immune system in the same way, and when one of these conditions is present in the body, the body becomes more susceptible to the other."*

This section could really be another entire book of its own, or really a whole *series* of books, but the goal is to introduce you to the idea of getting your home and office tested and remediating the mold as safely and effectively as possible. This should be done as soon as possible in your healing journey and is not to be thrown to the side. This can be accomplished with a simple at-home test called an ERMI, which can be ordered online OR as expensive as hiring experienced mold remediators and thoroughly checking the house (which is what I recommend).

If you live in an older home, have had water damage, possible slow leaks under sinks, roof issues, old office building…chances are, there's mold somewhere. Mold can be one of the most dangerous substances you breathe in and has been linked to MANY chronic illnesses.

e.) Supplementation

> *"Supplements can provide nutrients above and beyond what your diet is capable of providing. Their purpose is to help fill the voids."*

And boy, do we have voids in our diets today. Our soil isn't only depleted but our now food is too; it leaves us nutritionally depleted.

Supplementation is so important but often misunderstood. Proper supplementation is so personal and different for everybody. What's good for one person is not good for another. Taking more and more supplements isn't always better, either; it's just more.

Supplements can get unhealthy because taking too much of what you don't need can be toxic just like with anything else. Which is why you should always consult with a professional prior to taking any. There are also many gimmicky products out there that promise you the world and can be quite pricey. Some are good but some are plain 'ol bad. It's always best to take any and all supplements under the guidance of a practitioner. It's also important to choose high-quality products, some of which are only available from a practitioner.

How to maximize your supplement choices is to think first about your goal for taking them in the first place. Next is to figure out IF you have nutrient deficits. If you've been sick for a while, like many with chronic Lyme, then chances are you have depletions. Lastly, what body systems need support at the moment? When you have a plan and testing in place, you will get the most out of your supplementation choices! This is so very important and needed for speedy and efficient healing for anyone. Although supplementation is very individualized, there are some universal basics to always be utilizing for good foundational health and healing. They are as follows:

Gut Health Support

The human gut contains enough endotoxin, inflammatory mediators, and bacteria to kill the host many times over. A healthy functioning intestinal lining is our body's first line of defense against these dangerous agents. As we discussed earlier in chronic illness, toxins escaping from the gut lining release an inflammatory response, which then leads to further inflammation, tissue destruction, and production of cytokines and inflammatory mediators. Although a customized diet and lab testing to pinpoint the actual problems is hugely beneficial, there are a few main universal areas to focus on to encourage healing. The three fundamental aspects of gut health include the microbial population, physical structures and immune function. You can NOT expect gut restoration without supporting all three aspects of gut health. With that said, here are the three I recommend:

Soil-based probiotics: This is a pretty universal probiotic safe to take with a wide array of gut dysfunctions and sensitivities.

Although certain motility dysfunctions and disease cannot tolerate specific strains of probiotics and long term ill reactions can happen, you may also have specific sensitivities to certain strands and not know it. Soil-based probiotics will help encourage microbial diversity and growth of important health-promoting gut bacteria and at the same time being safe to take for many.

Carly's Top Picks:

- Megasporebiotic from Microbiome Labs

- Just Thrive

Mucosal Barrier Support: The goal is to rebuild and heal your mucosal barrier and leaky gut. The mucosal system is a very important part of the immune system. Mucus is extremely important and protective of us! It is the main interface between the human body and the outside world. The mucosal system contains 150 times more surface than skin which makes it one of the most important immune barriers. The health of the mucosa will determine how the body interacts with antigens. Oh boy! We know how this goes when dealing with Lyme. Supporting this system has been a game-changer for me and healing my leaky gut. It's a must! I have two products that I recommend here. They are:

Carly's Top Picks:

- Mega Mucosa from Microbiome Labs

- Support Mucosa from Biomatrix

Prebiotics: These guys don't get the attention that they deserve. This is the reinforcement of beneficial microbial changes created from our probiotics to create a strong and diverse microbiome. Prebiotics are non-digestible fibers that feed the bacteria living in your gut. The goal is to selectively feed the good bacteria not the bad and the problem here is that many prebiotics available on the market feed the good and the bad bacteria! For this reason, I only suggest one product:

Carly's Top Pick:

- MegaPrebiotic from Microbiome Labs

Digestion Support

This! This! This! This is a game-changer for most! Certain body systems slow down or take a back seat to other priority challenges when we are chronically ill. Our digestive function is one of them. A really popular phrase you may be familiar with is, "you are what you eat." and although it's true, it's not entirely true. You are what you digest! There are growing incidences of diseases that when traced back to the source, do appear to have links to nutrient malabsorption from lack of digestive enzymes. Enzymes' role in digestion act as a catalyst in speeding up specific life-preserving chemical reactions in the body. They assist in breaking down larger molecules into more easily absorbed particles that we need to thrive! If your body isn't producing adequate enzymes, then your absorption of nutrients may be affected, intestinal permeability will progress, hormone production will be affected, and much more. This is such an important piece of healing and cannot be overlooked. When challenged with Lyme, it can get tricky finding an enzyme that won't escalate your list of digestive symptoms. I have spent many years in trial and error in this department and lots of time studying. Here are my top picks and reasons why:

Carly's Top Picks:

- *Digestion GB from Pure Encapsulation*: Lyme and gallbladder issues are extremely common. Maybe not in the form of gallstones but gallbladder inflammation. This product is one that I'll probably be on the rest of my life. This enzyme formula supports healthy gallbladder function by utilizing bile salts, taurine, and herbal extracts all necessary for fat, carbohydrate, protein and to complement pancreatic enzyme activity.

- *Digestive Enzymes from Klaire Labs:* This lab has phenomenal products that I trust across the board but *this* particular product is amazing! I love that it is a basic formula without added ingredients. Less, more times than not is best! Many enzyme formulas contain HCL (Hydrochloric acid). I think HCL is a huge must-have in most maintenance plans POST healing. HCL in products can get tricky if you don't know what's truly going on in the intestines. There is so much information online stating how beneficial HCL is in curing leaky gut and for some this may be true but for most, it's not. HCL can be very dangerous to use if you don't know how to use it properly and always under the guidance of a professional. This did more damage than good for me. HCL is contraindicated with certain infections and can actually feed them. For this reason alone, I strictly only use plain enzyme formulas minus HCL until a certain level of recovery has happened. This formula is a safe and effective product that I use in my practice and personally used for years.

Immune Support

The goal is to equip your body with the tools it needs to fight and thrive! Immune system support is one powerful way to do this. This is so important in preparing the body for a healing protocol. It's never a good idea to throw any kind of medicine (natural *or* conventional) at a chronically ill individual. This is like throwing fuel in the fire, especially if you have chronic Lyme. In my personal experience, many times could have been saved had I known this simple truth. My body was too overwhelmed (with pathogenic infections, low nutrient stores, imbalanced metabolic system, overwhelmed liver and lymphatic system) and burdened and although I may have needed the medicine or herbs at the time, my body couldn't handle it and I always ended up sicker. Sicker with what I thought was horrific die-off reactions (but really I was just having a bad reaction and my body couldn't handle any kind of medicine or herbs). My body didn't have the tools to handle it. My minerals were tanked and my liver was overwhelmed. Replenishing the body's vitamins and minerals for a few weeks to a month *prior* to your healing protocol is so important! I use lots of high-quality sourced food-grade vitamins and minerals. Most with chronic illness have very sensitive systems and can't handle many synthetic forms.

I hear so often, "Increase your vitamin D and C to support your immune system. Or better yet, take zinc!" I think that is great advice and really important for immune function, but your immune system isn't a single entity. It's a system and requires balance and harmony from the whole body in order for it to function properly! Overwhelming the immune system when you have a chronic illness is *not* a good thing and can backfire in the form of heightening sensitivities and Lyme symptoms, but there are a few things I've found effective and only *after* those other lifestyle adjustments are made, which is why this section is placed where it is. Diet, detoxification, lifestyle and removing the toxins from our environment *prior* to supplementing for our immune function is the key to success here. I've also found that only using food grade products versus synthetic was hugely successful for me and most of my clients. Why would this make sense? Simple… Here's why:

- Synthetic minerals may not be excreted right away

- Synthetic vitamins do not contain trace minerals

- Synthetic vitamins can eventually become toxic

The body excretes natural vitamins while synthetic vitamins get stored in the liver as substances that can be toxic to the body. The body utilizes only what it needs from organic food-grade vitamins. I'm going to be short and sweet here. I'm not big on synthetic vitamins. For this reason alone, my list of support here is short as there aren't many good high quality sourced food-grade, multi-vitamins and supplements.

Carly's Top Picks:

SuperFood Plus from Dr. Schulze: As I mentioned earlier, our food and environment leave us nutrient depleted. I've been using this product for years to supplement the missing links. Remember, this is a food-grade product and your body will take and leave what it needs without added toxicity. In my opinion, food grade products are superior to synthetic! This contains 15 of the world's most powerful superfoods. My go-to for years as well as the number one product I use with most of my clients and family members.

Super-C from Dr. Schulze: This food grade vitamin C complex is life-changing. During leaky gut healing, ascorbic acid found in synthetic supplementation can be extremely aggravating to a delicate stomach lining. I always just assumed I couldn't tolerate vitamin C. Not the case! I couldn't tolerate the synthetic form of it as ascorbic acid.

Bermuda Triangle Support

Liver, Thyroid and Adrenals

These three organs as we've already extensively described as the Bermuda triangle are so important to prioritize as part of your base foundation of health. Also as we've discussed, you really can't support one and not the other for an effective long-term out-come. These organs are all intricately connected and depend on the function of the other. If you have one down, you know the other two are with it. If you support one, you need to support the other; they all depend on each other. Luckily, they all thrive on certain similar supplements for that reason.

The thyroid is the first organ that suffers during illness out of the entire body. The thyroid affects every single cell function in the body! Many with Lyme may not know that they do indeed have a thyroid component to their symptom storm. Many of the products we've already posted above will benefit these organs as well but for additional support, there is:

Carly's Top Picks:

- Endozin from Klaire Labs

- Selenium from Pure Encapsulations

- Milk Thistle from Jarrow Formulas

- Raw Dandelion Tea from Starwest Botanicals

- Liquid Vitamin D from Pure Encapsulations

- Magnesium Glycinate from Pure Encapsulations

f.) Cleaning Out The Oral Metals and Infections

"A healthy mouth may help you ward off medical disorders"

If you're anything like me, you may be wondering where in the world to start here. I started by changing my dentist! Does anyone know what a holistic or biological dentist is? They recognize and are trained in holistic health care. They recognize the mouthbody connection and uphold that in their dental practice.

"Holistic dentistry, also referred to as biological dentistry, is an alternative approach that focuses on the use of non-toxic restorative materials for dental work and emphasizes the unrecognized impact that dental toxins and dental infections may have on a person's overall health."

These dentists can be harder to come by but are in most states now! And drum roll please................most accept insurance!!!!! If you're used to visiting alternative or specialized health care practitioners, you are used to them not prescribing to insurance. This was a treat for my family. And, yes, even my children now see my biologic dentist.

The removal of these highly toxic fillings should not be done without safety measures in place. They should only be removed safely with a certified technician. The two biggest exposure risks with mercury fillings are when getting them implanted and then extracted. To lower the risk of mercury exposure, your certified dentist will have a high-volume evacuator and provide you with an alternative source of air, use of a dental dam, and have an air purification system in place. I was terrified to get this done but it was actually no big deal! This was a one-hour appointment to remove all three of my amalgam fillings and replace them with safe alternatives. I don't remember having any immediate health benefits but since then, my health recovery has progressed.

How do you know you have cavitation? My holistic dentist used a 3D cone beam scan and my surgeon used a CT scan. The cavitation appears as a shadow on the scan and can be missed by doctors that are not familiar with them. Choosing an oral surgeon took a lot of research on my part. It turns out that these surgeries have an extremely high recurrence rate when done improperly. After much research, I decided to go with Dr. Nunnally in Texas, which was a distant trip for me but worth it in my opinion. This choice was based on long-term success rates, cost, and practice. Many cavitation surgeries have a high recurrence rate because they aren't closed and cleaned up properly and the immune system isn't prepared appropriately. Dr. Nunnally uses Vit C IV drips for three days, ozone, platelets and stem cells to fill in the surgical spaces. The recovery period has been amazing with very little pain and swelling!

I think cavitation surgery is a very personal decision and one that can be incredibly beneficial. In my experience, individuals choose this only after many other health attempts have failed. This may or may not be your root cause but one thing is for sure, cavitations are a burden on the immune system which negatively affects the entire system. Amalgams are an easier resolution with a simple in-office usually insurance covered visit. There is no reason anyone should be keeping amalgam fillings in their mouth when there are perfectly safe alternatives to replace them with.

Now that we overhauled our diets to aid our recovery and limit our body's inflammatory burden, we've decreased our stress levels, are now getting high-quality sleep, exercising moderately, detoxing regularly, and supplementing our body with lots of gut healing and raw organic food-grade vitamins and minerals, we are now most likely gaining the benefits of lesser or eliminated symptoms. DO NOT be fooled though! Many may believe this is the answer as their fogs are lifting and the symptoms dwindling away. Remember, the goal is to feel better as soon as possible and eliminate the body's burdens. That was the goal of phase 1.

This is hopefully the case for you if you are following through completely. This is not the answer though! We still need to go in and clear out the infections and internal burdens for your long term health. Otherwise, you will need to sustain this very intense lifestyle that is just not feasible forever and risk the possibility of further disease. Hopefully by this point, we have our functional lab test results and can transition to phase 2!

PHASE 2

Kill And Re-Build

This is where the magic happens! This is also where the rubber meets the road. Lyme and other autoimmune illnesses may come in quietly but they don't leave quietly. Exiting chronic illness is no walk in the park and if you were to have some unpleasant experiences then this is usually the time. My experience in reducing my pathogenic load was not easy. My body was fighting active parasites, Borrelia, Bartonella EBV, yeast infections, H pylori, and probably more that I wasn't aware of. On top of all of that, once the pathogens start to die off, they let off a heavy burden of toxins and metals, creating what most know as the "herx" or the Jarisch Herxheimer Reaction. Not an easy thing to go through for most but my program is set up to absolutely minimize this experience. Having a strong and healthy body is the key to success here! By 100% adhering and completing phase 1, we minimize the effects in phase 2. Ever wonder why SO many people take antibiotics or herbal protocols for SO long and still not better afterward? This is why! A strong body with open detoxification pathways WILL work for YOU. period. Our bodies are capable of healing with proper tools in place. This phase usually lasts about 90 days with Lyme disease. That's right. 90 days on top of phase 1. Some of these infections can take some time to adequately clear up as some have specific life cycles, and parasites *do* lay eggs, which may not be eradicated in the first month or two of taking herbals. I know, insert gross emoji here.

a.) Why Natural Medicine?

My experience with treating my Lyme led me to what I do today. My personal experience with antibiotics was not successful and really made other issues more problematic for me. For this reason and many more, I choose a more natural holistic approach to healing Lyme.

Why I and other Lyme doctors, such as Dr. Rawls, believe antibiotics are not the best choice for Lyme:

1. Borrelia the infection that causes Lyme disease is a corkscrew shape that can bore deep into the tissues.

2. Borrelia can create cysts that are resistant to antibiotics.

3. Antibiotics can complicate stealth microbial coinfections.

4. Certain infections can become resistant to antibiotics.

5. Antibiotics can suppress your immune function.

6. Borrelia can create biofilms.

7. Antibiotics kill the good bacteria as well as the bad.

8. We don't have a cure yet.

Lyme isn't just about the Lyme and as I stated at the beginning of the book, disease is never just about the disease. Long term chronic Lyme disease is a much different beast from acute Lyme infection. Antibiotics show great clinical results with early detection but late-stage Lyme does not.

From the words of Dr. Rawls MD:

"As I came to know the microbe better, I began to understand why antibiotics are not necessarily a good treatment for chronic Lyme disease. Though some people do overcome Lyme disease with antibiotics, it doesn't occur consistently enough to be considered reliable. To date, no clinical studies have shown benefit from long-term antibiotic therapy for chronic Lyme disease." He then goes on to state that, *"I also met numerous people who had undergone 6-9 months of intravenous (IV) antibiotic therapy, only to be right back where they started within a couple of months of finishing the antibiotics."*

Ugh, to antibiotic or not to antibiotic...that is the question. That is usually the *big* question most struggle with once diagnosed with late-stage Lyme disease. That was my big question and I spent a good month researching doctors, pros and cons of different therapies and success rates and what I found were that the options in front of me were overwhelming! From Rife machines to drinking turpentine to months hooked up to IV antibiotic therapy. What I also found was that no two people seem to get out of Lyme the same, it takes a very long time to heal and will cost me oodles of money. Oh, have I mentioned insurance doesn't cover Lyme care? Insert emoji eye roll.

I ended up trying everything, including the kitchen sink...

- Antibiotics

- Herbs

- Long term liquid fasting

- Rife machine

- Hydrotherapy

- Blood Ozone

- IV therapy

- Hydrogen peroxide

This may seem like a lot but when you're desperate to heal and feel better you'll do and try just about anything to feel better. I get asked quite a lot how I healed my Lyme and I have to say it wasn't one thing that did it. Everything on that list is part of my progression to health and got me to where I am currently. Did I have to do it all? Probably not as I don't find most of them necessary knowing what I know now. I will say, my favorite and most effective therapy was the MOST expensive (of course). When my pain grew bad enough and I found myself enduring daily fevers and mostly bedridden with three small kids at home, my desperation took over. So I decided to travel to an intensive month-long IV clinic. This was one of the hardest decisions I've had to make to this date. The thought of leaving my three small children and husband for a whole month was awful but I knew in my heart it would be ok.

My symptoms were coming at alarming rates and some of which

got me in the ER routinely. It was no way to live and I wasn't getting the medical help I needed in my state. During my stay at the clinic, they had me doing daily blood ozone, hydrogen peroxide and vitamin IV. It was here that I also started heavy metal detoxing and utilizing light therapy. The Herx symptoms were pretty brutal and kept up for a few months after my return home but I got through it. It didn't do the job though as I was still sick. Insert cry emoji. I was not bedridden anymore but still experiencing many Lyme symptoms.

After paying tens of thousands of dollars on a Lyme protocol YOU SHOULD FEEL AMAZING! This is when I found myself back in school. I decided it was time to only invest in myself. Enough was enough. As I watched my friends I've now made in the Lyme arena continue to suffer as well, I just knew a change needed to be made. There had to be a better way! Please know that you don't need to spend tens of thousands and suffer needlessly. During my few years of trial and error and countless doctors, it became very clear that maybe I was looking at this all wrong. I was so focused on killing the Lyme and its posse that maybe I was the one keeping me sick? This is when I started to seek out as many people as possible who've recovered and learn how they did it. I found the common link was focusing on the gut, detoxification and lifestyle. It wasn't just boatloads of antibiotics, herbs and medicines. Interesting as this is also the focus I began learning in my new endeavor to become certified as a functional diagnostic nutritional practitioner. A total body approach!

We've made a list of why antibiotics may not be the best approach to healing chronic Lyme, now let's look at some very compelling reasons Dr. Rawls makes on why to choose herbs:

1. Herbs provide a wide spectrum of antimicrobial properties.

2. Using multiple herbs together is synergistic.

3. Herbs are inherently safe.

4. Herbs enhance immune functions.

5. Herbs support a balanced microbiome.

6. Herbs help the body deal with biofilms and cyst forms.

7. Herbs provide a wide spectrum of other benefits.

Recovery from a chronic illness is truly complex and requires an individualized plan as we've clearly shown. Let's take a peek at a few very comprehensive and effective herbal programs that are time tested, affordable, and met with great success! But first, a few reminders as you set out on this new phase of healing:

- Do not stop detoxing! Increase if needed!

- Do not stop exercising no matter how tired you are!

- Eliminate any emotional trauma with a professional!

- Detox!

- Sleep hard and long at night!

- Now is NOT the time to cheat on the eating plan and alcohol!

- Detox!

- Stay very hydrated!

- Keep taking your phase 1 supplements!

- Detox!

- Spiritual enrichment!

- Detox!

- Did I mention detox?

Ok then, now that we have an understanding of how to get the maximum out of this process, let's get started on phase 2! But, just so we are clear, **detox as much as possible and utilize ALL the methods.** Just to refresh your memory, here are my favorite and most effective forms of detoxing:

- Salt flushing

- Lymphatic massage

- Hot and cold hydrotherapy

- Dry skin brushing

- Professional colonics

- Herbs

- Coffee enemas

- Epsom salt baths

- Acupuncture

- Cupping

- Chiropractic care

Just keep rotating the different forms of detoxing and continue to utilize the colon clearing ones as much as needed until symptoms start to disappear. You'll be *so* happy you did!

Please keep in mind that no medicine, supplement, or herb will work unless you are doing all the other necessary things in conjunction! Healing chronic illness is a very complex and comprehensive process.

Carly's Top Picks:

Biocidin, Biotonic, and Oliverix from Biobotanical Research: These are a trio that needs to be taken together for efficiency. They are a power player in Lyme, parasite, yeast and viral healing.

- *Biocidin:* Over 30 years of clinical testing and effectiveness, leading nutritional support by many practitioners, botanicals to assist detoxification pathways, research indicates addressing biofilms associated with pathogens.

- *Biotonic:* This is a supportive formula that complements Biocidin. I see many practitioners using Biocidin alone with little success. This complementary formula supports the liver, adrenals, GI tract, and will help strengthen the body's defense systems when herbs are used for long periods of time.

- *Olivirex:* This very potent olive leaf extract is a power-house. This will help support the clearance of toxins from the body!

The Buhner protocol: This is an amazing doctor online that many have tremendous success with! His protocol is very straightforward and with little products that can be purchased in bulk and put together yourself if needed. His three core herbs are pretty universal and used in many other protocols. They are time tested and commonly known for eradicating Lyme and its Co-infections. They are as follows:

- Japanese knotweed root (Polygonum Cuspidatum)

- Cats Claw (Uncaria Tomentosa)

- Andrographis (Andrographis Paniculata)

My simple recipe: Simple way to get the maximum for the minimum cost. I buy them in bulk from a high-quality source and mix them in a jar. This can be placed into gel caps or simply spooned into a liquid to be drunk which is what I chose to do for ease of use. This doesn't taste the best but it is tolerable.

The herbs are as follows:

- Black Walnut ½ cup

- Sweet Wormwood ½ cup

- Olive Leaf ½ cup

- Cat's Claw ½ cup

- Pau D' Arco ¼ cup

All of these programs I've stated above are broad spectrum and are used to work on multiple pathogen eradication protocols. With that will come a more intense healing journey as the level of pathogens dying off will be beyond what our detoxification organs may be able to withstand, which will contribute to your level of Herx reaction. Because of this, a binder is necessary to mop up the mess we are clearing out.

Carly's Top Picks:

G.I. Detox from Biobotanical Research: This is a full spectrum binder that supports enhanced clearance for microbial balance in the GI Tract. This will also assist in biofilm removal.

When taking herbs, always, and I repeat, ALWAYS titrate your way up to the maximum suggested dose on the bottle or by your practitioner. I always suggest starting one at a time and at the minimum dosages to avoid any complications.

Well, well, well, look where we are. That wasn't terrible, was it?! Believe me, it can be this basic when you look at the whole picture. The first few weeks of adjusting to herbs are usually the most challenging but after you get past the adjustment period skies the limit. This is when I really started to feel good. I'm so excited for you and can't wait to hear about your recovery journey. Now let's get into the fun part...maintenance and recovery!

PHASE 3

Maintenance and Recovery

I get asked a lot if I'm healed from Lyme disease. This is a tough question to answer! Mostly because there's no way to test if you truly are healed and unfortunately, testing is very questionable and unreliable. Two of the most utilized tests from conventional medical doctors that are initially run for Lyme Disease diagnosis are called the Western Blot and Elisa. These tests can miss up to 60% of well-defined Lyme disease cases. The antibodies your body creates to fight the infection may not ever go away, but that doesn't mean your infection is still alive and active!

On another note, those antibodies will NOT protect you from another future Lyme infection so prevention is always key. I think answering this question is very personal and unique to everyone. Am I back to my old full marathon running self? No. But, I'm happy to report that I live my life now mostly symptom-free, I'm endurance running again (half marathons), running my own thriving business, and have full energy throughout the day. No more brain fog, afternoon naps, headaches, limb numbness, body pain, daily digestive issues, nor sleep issues. I feel better than I have in years! I will always be following some sort of maintenance plan and always have my thoughts on my *continued* healing. This is *so* important to remember!

I find many wanting to jump back into their old ways too soon after recovery and it always seems to backfire. That's why chronic illness is usually considered to be a lifestyle illness. We don't get sick overnight and we don't heal overnight.

To summarize what we've already revealed; these unhealthy life-style choices year after year seem to be the contributing factors in chronic illness in the form of stress, poor diet, external and internal stress, unhealthy and toxic relationships, substance abuse, and over and under physical exercise.

Chronic illness has the potential to truly be life-changing when we have no choice but to face ourselves. Making the long-term changes may be challenging for you; some were for me! Know you are worth it! If you've made it to this point, you've most likely already found much healing and symptom recovery but healing from Lyme and other chronic illnesses can take time. Which is why it's important to **stay the course** and continue to support your body.

Here's what I recommend for on-going supplement support:

1. Gut support:

   • Megasporebiotic from Microbiome Labs

   • Megaprebiotic from Microbiome Labs

   • Megamucosa from Microbiome Labs

2. Digestion support:

   • Digestion Enzymes Ultra with Betaine HCL from Pure Encapsulations

3. Immune system support:

   • Superfood 100 from Dr. Schulze

- Super C from Dr. Schulze

- Liquid Vitamin D

Never stop taking personal internal inventories. Our bodies talk to us through our physical bodies. Pay attention to it going forward. This is key for long term health and avoiding falling into old bad habits and patterns that got us sick to begin with.

My journey has shown me that so much growth and unexpected blessings can come from the darkest of places. I've grown tremendously in so many ways that I know for sure wouldn't have, had I not been sick. I am forever grateful for the spiritual, emotional and physical place I am today. Lyme and chronic illness isn't a death sentence but truly can make your life miserable with their unrelenting symptoms if you allow it. Don't let it control your life one more day...***act now!***

I've found success in numbers. We aren't meant to do this alone. I've met some of the most amazing people on my journey. From some of the most amazing doctors, one of whom prayed with me, to friends I'm now forever bonded with by a commonality through disease and healing. Open your heart to the amazing opportunities this journey may take you! Lean in and let it all in. Know that you are never alone.

I've walked the walk and fully understand the fear, confusion, anxiety, and sadness illness can provide. Reach out to me, I want to hear from you!

My program is available all over the world! Know that healing can be done without professional guidance but personalized assistance will not only save you time but ultimately money spent in the long haul. Functional lab testing is truly amazing and the information gained will benefit you immensely. Knowledge truly is power!

It truly is unfortunate that in today's world, we have a disease more prevalent than AIDS, West Nile, and the Avian Flu combined, and still no significant medical attention. BUT, we do have answers for relief and healing in the functional healthcare system. We have answers on how to provide your body with the tools to work on your behalf! If you're stuck in a tug-of-war with sickness and healing, then it is time to try something different. Don't EVER stop seeking answers! Don't settle! I've provided you with a very detailed and lengthy guide on how YOU can personally navigate and take back your healing journey.

"As I sit here in this dark room all alone, tears dripping down my face, IV's in my arms, fear pulsating through my body, I can't help but wonder, will this be my magic treatment? Will I finally be healed? Why does no one hear me and understand how bad this disease really is?"

I hear you, I see you, I understand and I know that you can be free from the symptom-hell you may be entangled with.

Today is Day One of the rest of your life. Don't let your illness rule you one more day!

Your friend, in sickness and in health,

Carly

About the Author

Carly Herter is a certified and trained Functional Diagnostic Nutritional Practitioner, holistic health coach, and most recently received her board certification from the AADP (American Association of Drugless Practitioners).

She has extensive experience in working with clients all over the world, focusing mostly on autoimmunity and chronic late-stage Lyme disease. Her success in the field comes not only from her unique training but also from her extensive personal experience with multiple chronic illnesses. Carly never tires of staying up to date with research, education, and certifications as well as collaborating with other influencers and practitioners.

Carly works out of her home and spends most of her time with her three young children and husband in a small town on the coast of New Hampshire. She enjoys long-distance running, reading, cooking, entertaining, crafting, and spending time with her family. After experiencing years of trial and error, lack of medical support and escalating sickness, Carly is determined and passionate to assist those still stuck in the merry-go-round of darkness associated with autoimmunity and Lyme disease.

REFERENCES

The Roots of it All

1. Epidemiology and estimated population burden of selected autoimmune diseases in the United States. DL Jacobson et al. Clin Immunol Immunopathol. 1997 Sep. https://Pubmed.ncbi.nlm.nih.gov/9281381/

2. The gut-brain axis: historical reflections. Ian Miller. www.ncbi.nlm.nih.gov/pmc/articles/pmc6225396

3. The gut microbiome: Relationships with disease and opportunities for therapy. Juliana Durack et al. J Exp Med. 2019. https://pubmed.ncbi.nlm.nih.gov/30322864/

4. Role of intestinal microbiota and metabolites on gut homeostasis and human diseases. Lan Lin et al. BMC Immunol. 2017. https://pubmed.ncbi.nlm.nih.gov/28061847/

5. Human Intestinal Microbiota: Interaction between parasites and the host immune response. Oswaldo

Partida-Rodriguez et al. Arch Med Res. 2017 Nov. https://pubmed.ncbi.nlm.nih.gov/29290328/

Section 1: The Cause

1. Cause and effect. https://www.nature.com/articles/nrmicro1437

2. Lifestyle medicine: the future of chronic disease management. Kushner RF, et al. Curr Opin Endocrinol Diabetes Obes. 2013. https://pubmed.ncbi.nlm.nih.gov/23974765/

3. Why physiology is critical to the practice of medicine: A 40-year personal perspective. Martin J. Tobin. Clin chest Med. 2019 Jun. https://pubmed.ncbi.nlm.nih.gov/31078207/

4. Case of iatrogenic botulism after botulinotherapy in clinical in clinical practice. R A lbatullin et al. Ter Arkh. 2018. https://pubmed.ncbi.nlm.nih.gov/30701823/

5. Botulinum Toxin Deaths: What is the Fact? Omprakash HM and Rajendran SC. https://ncbi.nlm.nih.gov/pmc/articles/PMC2840902/

6. Is Botox Poisonous? Here's what you need to know. Emily Cronkleton May 2018. Medically reviewed by Catherine Hannan M.D. https://www.healthline.com/health/botox-poison

7. Natural compounds and their analogues as potent antidotes against the most poisonous bacterial toxin. Kruti

B Patel et al. Appl Environ Microbiol. 2018. https://pubmed.ncbi.nlm.nih.gov/30389764/

8. Serious and Long-Term Adverse Events Associated with the Therapeutic and Cosmetic Use of Botulinum Toxin. Yiannakopoulou E. https://www.karger.com/article/fulltext/370245

9. Injections of Clostridium Botulinum neurotoxin A may cause thyroid complications in predisposed persons based on molecular mimicry with thyroid autoantigens. Edvina Gregoric et al. Endocrine. 2011 Feb. https://pubmed.ncbi.nlm.nih.gov/21061092/

10. Botox makes unnerving journey into our nervous system. April 16, 2015. https://www.sciencedaily.com/releases/2015/04/150416094051.htm

11. Considering the immune response to Botulinum Toxin. Jeff Critchfield. Nov 2002. https://www.researchgate.net/publication/10915300_considering_the_immune_response_to_botulinum_toxin

12. Cosmetic injection of Botulinum toxin unmasking subclinical Myasthenia Gravis: A case report and literature review. Timmermans G. Depierreux F. Wang F. Hansen I. Maquet P. https://www.karger.com/article/fulltext/502350

13. Serious and long-term adverse events associated with the therapeutic and cosmetic use of botulinum toxin. Eugenia Yiannakopoulou. Pharmacology. 2015. https://

pubmed.ncbi.nlm.nih.gov/25613637/

14. Clinical analysis of 86 botulism cases caused by cosmetic injection of botulinum toxin (BoNT) Lili Bai et al. Medicine (Baltimore). 2018 Aug. https://pubmed.ncbi.nlm.nih.gov/30142749/

15. Poisoning with botulinum neurotoxin—diagnostic difficulties. S Grygorczuk et al. Pol Merkur Lekarski. 2000 Aug. https://pubmed.ncbi.nlm.nih.gov/1081329/

16. Living with the past: evolution, development, and patterns of disease. Peter D Gluckman et al. Science. 2004. https://pubmed.ncbi.nlm.nih.gov/5375258/

17. Prioritising risk pathways of complex human diseases based on functional profiling. Yan Li et al. Eur J Hum Genet. 2013 Jun. https://pubmed.ncbi.nlm.nih.gov/23047740/

18. Integrated chronic disease prevention and control: Community based programmes. Https://who.int/chp/about/integrated_cd/en/index2.html

19. Latest APA survey reveals deepening concerns about connection between chronic disease and stress. 2012. https://www.apa.org/news/press/releases/2012/01/chronic-disease

20. How do stress and inflammation contribute to chronic disease? https://ifm.org/news-insights/inflam-stress-inflammation-contribute-chronic-disease/

21. Nutritional keys for intestinal barrier modulation. Stefania De Santis, Elisabetta Cavalcanti and Marcello Chieppa. https://www.ncbi.nlm.nih.gov/pmc/articles/PMC4670985/

22. Neurodegenerative disease: Improving outcomes through nutrition. https://ifm.org/news-insights/neuro-slowing-neurodegeneration-with-nutrition/

23. The Power of Functional Nutrition. https://ifm.org/news-insights/power-functional-nutrition-2/

24. Global diets link environmental sustainability and human health. David Tilman et al. Nature. 2014. https://pubmed.ncbi.nlm.nih.gov/25383533/

25. The anti-inflammatory effects of exercise: mechanisms and implications for the prevention and treatment of disease. Michael Gleeson et al. Nat Rev Immunol. 2011. https://pubmed.ncbi.nlm.gov/21818123/

26. Overtraining, Exercise, and Adrenal Insufficiency. Ka Brooks et al. J Nov Physiother. 2013. https://pubmed.ncbi.nlm.nih.gov/23667795/

27. The balance between food and dietary supplements in the general population. Dr. Marleen AH Lentjes, Senior Research Nutritionist. https://www.ncbi.nlm.nih.gov/pmc/articles/PMC6366563/

28. What you need to know about dietary supplements. https://www.fda.gov/food/buy-store-serve-safe-food/

what-you-need-know-about-dietary-supplements

29. Statement from FDA Commissioner Scott Gottlieb,
M.D. on the agency's new efforts to strengthen regulation of dietary supplements by modernizing and re-
forming FDA's oversight. 2/11/2019. www.fda.gov/
news-events/press-anouncements/statement-fda-commis-
sioner-scott-gottlieb-md-agencys-new-efforts-strengthen-
regulation-dietary

30. Studying how pathogens cause disease. https://
www.fda.gov/drugs/news-events-human-drugs/
studying-how-pathogens-cause-disease

31. Viral Infections and Autoimmune Disease: Roles
of LCMV in Delineating Mechansims of Immune
Tolerance. Georgia Fousteri et al. Viruses. 2019. https://
pubmed.ncbi.nlm.nih.gov/31546586/

32. Infections as triggers of flares in systemic autoimmune
diseases: novel innate immunity mechanisms. Honorio
Torres-Aguilar et al. Curr Opin Rheumatol. 2019 Sep.
https://pubmed.ncbi.nlm.nih.gov/31135383/

33. From autoinflammation to autoimmunity: old and re-
cent findings. Francesco Caso et al. Clin Rheumatol.
2018 Sep. https://pubmed.ncbi.nlm.nih.gov/30014358/

34. Alcohol and Toxicity. Ivan Rusyn and Ramon
Bataller. https://www.ncbi.nlm.nih.gov.pmc/articles/
PMC3959903/

35. Metabolic consequences of alcohol ingestion. TJ Peters et al. Novartis Found Symp. 1998. https://pubmed.ncbi.nlm.nih.gov/9949785/

36. Vitiligo and Hashimoto's thyroiditis: Autoimmune diseases linked by clinical presentation, biochemical commonality, and autoimmune/oxidative stress-mediated toxicity pathogensis. Dongmei Li et al. Med Hypotheses. 2019 Jul. https://pubmed.ncbi.nlm.gov/31203913/

37. Chronic illness associated with mold and mycotoxins: Is naso-sinus fungal biofilm the culprit? Joseph H. Brewer, Jack D. Thrasher, and Dennis Hooper. https://www.ncbi.nlm.nih.gov/pmc/articles/PMC3920250/

38. What primary physicians should know about environmental causes of illness. William J. Rea, MD. 2009. https://journalofethics.ama-assn.org/article/what-primary-physicians-should-know-about-environmental-causes-illness/2009-06

39. Oral health: A window to your overall health. Mayo Clinic Staff. https://www.mayoclinic.org/healthylifestyle/adult-health/in-depth/dental/art-20047475

Section 2: The Effect

1. Leaky gut: mechanisms, measurement and clinical implications in humans. Michael Camilleri. Gut. 2019 Aug. https://pubmed.ncbi.nlm.nih.gov/31076401/

2. Retinoic Acid, Leaky Gut, and Autoimmune Diseases.

Leila Abdelhamid et al. Nutrients. 2018. https://pubmed.ncbi.nlm.nih.gov/30081517/

3. The intestinal microbiota, a leaky gut, and abnormal immunity in kidney disease. Hans-Joachim Anders et al. Kidney Int. 2013 Jun. https://pubmed.ncbi.nlm.nih.gov/30081517/

4. Many recovering from addiction have chronic health problems, diminished quality of life. March 21, 2019. https://sciencedaily.com/releases/2019/03/190321092201.htm

5. Exercise-induced stress behavior, gut-microbiota-brain axis and diet: a systemic review for athletes. Allison Clark et al. J Int Soc sports Nutr. 2016. https://pubmed.ncbi.nlm.nih.gov/27924137/

6. Physiology of intestinal absorption and secretion. Pawel R. Kiela, DVM, PhD and Fayez K. Ghishan, MD. https://www.ncbi.nlm.nih.gov/pmc/articles/pmc4956471/

7. The spectrum of small intestinal bacterial overgrowth (SIBO). Eamonn M M Quigley. Curr Gastroenterol Rep. 2019. https://pubmed.ncbi.nlm.nih.gov/30645678/

8. Brain fogginess, gas and bloating: a link between SIBO, probiotics and metabolic acidosis. Satish S C Rao et al. Clin Transl Gastroenterol. 2018. https://pubmed.ncbi.nlm.nih.gov/29915215/

9. IgA nephropathy and infections. Cristiana Rollino et al. J Nephrol. 2016 Aug. https://pubmed.ncbi.nlm.nih.gov/26800970/

10. Gastrointestinal symptoms of Lyme Disease. Dr. Todd Maderis. https://drtoddmaderis.com/gastrointesinal-lyme-disease

11. The metabolic syndrome is associated with complicated gallstone disease. Naim Ata, MD, Metin Kucukazman, MD and Yasar Nazligul, MD. https://www.ncbi.nlm.nih.gov/pmc/articles/PMC3115009/

12. Metabolic syndrome and gallstone disease. Li-Ying Chen, Qiao-Hua Qiao and Li-Zheng Fang. https://www.ncbi.nlm.nih.gov/pmc/articles/PMC3422804/

13. A systemic Review of Biological Mechanisms of Fatigue in Chronic Illness. Lea Ann Matura et al. Biol Res Nurs. 2018 Jul. https://pubmed.ncbi.nlm.nih.gov/2954006/

14. Human digestion—a processing perspective. Mike Boland. J Sci Food Agric. 2016 May. https://pubmed.ncbi.nlm.nih.gov/26711173/

15. The digestive system: linking theory and practice. T Hoyle. Br. Nurs. 1997 Dec 11-1998 Jan 7. https://pubmed.ncbi.nlm.nih.gov/9470654/

16. The Influence of the Gut Microbiome on Cancer, Immunity, and Cancer Immunotherapy. Vancheswaran Gopalakrishnan et al. Cancer Cell. 2018. https://

pubmed.ncbi.nlm.nih.gov/29634945/

17. Gastroparesis: Medical and Therapeutic Advances. Christopher M Navas et al. Dig Dis Sci. 2017 Sep. https://pubmed.ncbi.nlm.nih.gov/28721575/

18. Epidemiology and pathophysiology of Gastroparesis. Baha Moshiree et al. Gastrointest Endosc Clin N Am. 2019 Jan. https://pubmed.ncbi.nlm.nih.gov/30396519/

19. Mast Cell Activation Syndrome. https://lymedisease.org/mast-cell-activation-syndrome/

20. The Multifaceted Role of Mast Cells in Cancer: When do mast cells inhibit cancer proliferation, and when do they contribute to it? Jacob Schor, ND FABNO. Feb 2011 Vol. 3 issue 2. https://www.naturalmedicinejournal.com/journal/2011-02/multifaceted-role-mast-cells-cancer

21. Approaches to testing for food and chemical sensitivities. Bruce R Gordon. Otolaryngology Clin North Am. 2003 Oct. https://pubmed.ncbi.nlm.nih.gov/14743781/

22. Non-Ige-mediated gastrointestinal food allergy. Anna Nowak-Wegrzyn et al. J Allergy Clin Immunol. 2015 May. https://pubmed.ncbi.nlm.nih.gov/25956013/

23. Immune responses in the Liver. Paul Kubes et al. Annu Rev Immunol. 2018. https://pubmed.ncbi.nlm.nih.gov/29328785/

24. Liver abnormalities and endocrine diseases. Patrizia Burra. Best Pract Res Clin Gastroenterol. 2013 Aug.

https://pubmed.ncbi.nlm.nih.gov/24090942/

25. Studies on the functional relationship between thyroid, adrenal and gonadal hormones. Atsushi Tohei. J Reprod Dev. 2004 Feb. https://pubmed.ncbi.nlm.nih.gov/15007197/

26. Pathology of immune-mediated liver injury. Hans-peter Dienes et al. Dig Dis. 2010. https://pubmed.ncbi.nlm.nih.gov/20460891/

27. Dietary cholesterol does not break your heart but kills your liver. Gerhard P. Puschel, MD and Janin Henkel, PhD. https://www.ncbi.nlm.nih.gov/pmc/articles/PMC6726297/

28. The immune system and kidney disease: basic concepts and clinical implications. Christian Kurts et al. Nat Rev Immunol. 2013 Oct. https://pubmed.ncbi.nlm.nih.gov/24037418/

29. Emerging role of fecal microbiota therapy in the treatment of gastrointestinal and extra-gastrointestinal diseases. P C Konturek et al. J Physiol pharmacol. 2015 Aug. https://pubmed.ncbi.nlm.nih.gov/26348073/

30. Lymphatic System. https://my.clevelandclinic.org/health/articles/21199-lymphatic-system

Section 3: The Healing Solution

1. The growing trend of health coaches in team-based primary care training a multicenter pilot study. Nicole M

Gastala et al. Fam Med. 2018 Jul. https://pubmed.ncbi.nlm.nih.gov/30005115/

2. From complimentary to integrative medicine and health: Do we need a change in nomenclature? Dieter Melchart. Complement Med Res. 2018. https://www.karger.com/article/fulltext/488623

3. Treatment Interventions for the Management of Intestinal Permeability: A Cross-Sectional Survey of Complementary and Integrative Medicine Practitioners. Bradley Leech et all. J Altern Complement Med. 2019 Jun. https://pubmed.ncbi.nlm.nih.gov/31038350/

4. Investigation into complementary and integrative medicine practitioners' clinical experience of intestinal permeability: A cross-sectional survey. Bradley Leech et al. Complement Ther Clin Pract. 2018 May. https://pubmed.ncbi.nlm.nih.gov/29705456/

5. Social determinants and lifestyles: integrating environmental and public health perspectives. H Graham et al. Public Health. 2016 Dec.

6. The Clinical Application Value of Multiple Combination Food Intolerance Testing. Shudong Lin et al. Iran J Public Health. 2019 Jun. https://pubmed.ncbi.nlm.nih.gov/31341848/

7. Food Intolerance: Immune Activation Through Diet-associated Stimuli in Chronic Disease. Nicole Peitschmann. Altern Ther Health Med. Jul-Aug 2015.

https://pubmed.ncbi.nlm.nih.gov/26030116/

8. Alleviating gastro-intestinal symptoms and concerns by integrating patient-tailored complementary supportive cancer care. Eran Ben-Arye et al. Clin Nutr. 2015 Dec. https://pubmed.ncbi.nlm.nih.gov/25556349

9. Naturopathic Approaches to Irritable Bowel Syndrome-A Delphi Study. Joshua Z Goldenberg et al. J Altern Complement Med. 2019 Feb. https://pubmed.ncbi.nlm.nih.gov/30207740/

10. Diet, nutrition and the prevention of chronic diseases. Report of the joint WHO/FAO expert consultation. https://www.who.int/dietphysicalactivity/publications/trs916/summary/en/

11. Immune Suppression of IgG response against dairy proteins in major depression. Leszek Rudzki et al. BMC Psychiatry. 2017. https://pubmed.ncbi.nlm.nih.gov/28738849/

12. The Multiple pathways to autoimmunity. Argyrios N Theofilopoulos et al. Nat Immunol. 2017. https://pubmed.ncbi.nlm.nih.gov/28632714/

13. Multiplex polymerase chain reaction tests for detection of pathogens associated with gastroenteritis. Hongwei Zhang et al. Clin Lab Med. 2015 Jun. https://pubmed.ncbi.nlm.nih.gov/26004652/

14. Impact of Gastrointestinal Panel Implementation on

Health Care Utilization and Outcomes. Jordan E. Axelrad et al. J Clin Microbiol 2019. https://pubmed. ncbi.nlm.nih.gov/30651393/

15. Healthy diet could save $50 billion in health care costs. Brigham and Women's Hospital. December 17,2019. https://www.sciencedaily.comreleas-es/2019/12/191217141314.htm

16. Nutritional Protocol for the Treatment of Intestinal Permeability Defects and Related Conditions. Corey Resnick, ND. March 2010 Vol. 2 issue 3. https://www. naturalmedicinejournal.com/journal/2010-03/nutrition-al-protocol-treatment-intestinal-permeability-defects-and-related

17. Mycotoxins in Bovine Milk and Dairy Products: A Review. Tania Aparecida Becker-Algeri et al. J Food Sci. Mar 2016. https://pubmed.ncbi.nlm.nih.gov/26799355

18. Consumption of dairy products and the risk of breast cancer: a review of the literature. Patricia G Moorman et al. Am J clin Nutr. 2004 Jul. https://pubmed.ncbi.nlm. nih.gov/15213021/

19. Dairy cattle serum and milk factors contributing to the risk of colon and breast cancers. Harold Zur Hausen et al. Int J Cancer. 2015. https://pubmed.ncbi.nlm.nih. gov/25648405

20. Dairy: Do you really need it? https://www. nm.org/healthbeathealthy-tips/nutrition/

dairy-do-you-really-need-it

21. Problems digesting dairy products? https://
www.fda.gov/consumers/consumer-updates/
problems-digesting-dairy-products

22. How to boost your immune system. April 6, 2020.
https://www.health.harvard.edu/staying-healthy/
how-to-boost-your-immune-system

23. Why Americans Need Information on Dietary
Supplements. Johanna T Dwyer et al. J Nutr. 2018.
https://pubmed.ncbi.nlm.nih.gov/31505678/

24. Dietary Supplements. Patrick B Massey. Med Clin
North Am. 2002 Jan. https://pubmed.ncbi.nlm.nih.
gov/11795085/

25. Complimentary and integrative treatments: thyroid
disease. Jennifer E Rosen et al. Otolaryngology Clin
North Am. 2013 Jun. https://pubmed.ncbi.nlm.nih.
gov/23764819/

26. Leadership in global oral health. David M Williams
et al. J Dent. 2019 Aug. https://pubmed.ncbi.nih.
gov/31075367/

27. Evidence supporting a link between dental amalgams and
chronic illness, fatigue, depression, anxiety, and suicide.
Janet K Kern et al. Neuro Endocrinol Lett. 2014. https://
pubmed.ncbi.nlm.nih.gov/25617876

28. Oral inflammation and infection, and chronic

medical diseases: implications for the elderly. Frank A Scannapieco et al. Periodontal 2000. 2016 Oct. https://pubmed.ncbi.nlm.nih.gov/27501498/

29. Remission of aggressive autoimmune disease (dermato-myositis) with removal of infective jaw pathology and ozone case report. Robert Jay Rowen. Auto Immune Highlights. 2018. https://pubmed.ncbi.nlm.nih.gov/29959639/

30. Rantes and fibroblast growth factor 2 in jawbone cavitations: triggers for systemic disease? Johann Lechner et al. Int J Gen Med. 2013. https://pubmed.ncbi.nlm.nih.gov/23637551/

31. Estimation of cumulative number of post-treatment Lyme disease cases in the US, 2016 and 2020. Allison DeLong et al. BMC Public Health. 2019. https://pubmed.ncbi.nlm.nih.gov/31014314/

32. Lyme disease diagnosis and treatment: lessons from the AIDS epidemic. R B Stricker et al. Minerva Med. 2010 Dec. https://pubmed.ncbi.nlm.nih.gov/21196901/

33. Evaluation of natural and botanical medicines for activity against growing and non-growing forms of B. burgdor-feri. Jie Feng et al. Front Med (Lausanne). 2020. https://pubmed.ncbi.nlm.nih.gov/32154254/

34. The controversies, challenges and complexities of Lyme Disease: A narrative review. Marie Claire Van Hout. J Pharm Sci. 2018. https://pubmed.ncbi.nlm.nih.

gov/30458921/

35. Challenges in the Diagnosis and Treatment of Lyme Disease. Robert T Schoen. Curr RHeumatol Rep. 2020. https:// pubmed.ncbi.nlm.nih.gov/31912251/

36. Seven herbal medicines can kill Lyme disease bacteria in test tube. Feb 21, 2020. https://www.lymedisease.org/seven-herbals-kill-lyme-disease/

37. Lyme disease and the epistemic tensions of "medically unexplained illnesses". Abigail A Dumes. Med Anthropol. Aug-Sep 2020. https://pubmed.ncbi.nlm.nih.gov/31860363/

CPSIA information can be obtained
at www.ICGtesting.com
Printed in the USA
LVHW110512100221
678886LV00005B/484

9 781977 230607